D. Van Nostrand Company Regional Offices:
New York   Cincinnati

D. Van Nostrand Company International Offices:
London   Toronto   Melbourne

Published by D. Van Nostrand Company
135 West 50th Street, New York, N.Y. 10020

10 9 8 7 6 5 4 3 2 1

Preface

The need for greater emphasis on education in research to improve nursing practice was recognized by the Commission on Nursing Research of the American Nurses' Association in its guidelines published in 1976. The guidelines recommend that education in research on the undergraduate level provide an introduction to research, including a beginning experience in the research process. Education in research also should prepare the nurse to read research reports critically and provide an understanding of the rights and responsibilities of both participants and subjects in research.

It has been our experience that students exposed to the research process for the first time find that their learning is facilitated (and their anxiety reduced) when they are guided through the research process in a systematic, step-by-step manner and when opportunities are provided for the practical implementation of the research process inherent in preparing a research proposal.

This book is intended to provide basic nursing research principles and techniques. Included are step-by-step activities designed to help the beginning research student read research reports critically, prepare a nursing research proposal, and understand the proposal's relationship to a completed research report. No statistical background is required by the student.

Research proposals submitted by students in a basic nursing research class are presented as appendixes because they reflect the level of performance expected of the beginning researcher. The written report of the research study implementing the proposal of one of these beginning research students is also included.

Critical Reviewers

Barbara A. Backer, R.N., M.A., Herbert H. Lehman College
Virginia J. Harris, R.N., Ed.D., Temple University
Anne Kibrick, R.N., Ed.D., Boston State College
Ann F. Muhlenkamp, R.N., Ph.D., Arizona State University
Paulette Robischon, R.N., Ph.D., Herbert H. Lehman
  College
Theresa M. Valiga, R.N., Ed.M., Georgetown University
Jane H. White, R.N., Ph.D., George Mason University

Contents

Appendixes

Part 1

Becoming Acquainted with Nursing Research

The material in Chapter 1 is designed to acquaint you with the nature of research by introducing some basic concepts related to research in general and nursing research in particular. It also provides a brief overview of the historical development of nursing research in the United States.

1

The Nature of Research and Nursing Research

THIS chapter is designed to introduce you to nursing research by helping you understand some basic concepts related to the what and why of research in general, and nursing research in particular.

What Is Research?

Now that you are beginning your experience with research—particularly nursing research—it is important that you understand what research *is* and what research *is not*.

If you are like many other people, you probably associate the word research with experiments conducted in the laboratory on various animals, or with the discovery of new drugs or treatment methods in medical science. You may also associate research with the scientific experiments conducted on the moon during the past years.

What Research Is

In reality, the word research has many different meanings and broad applications; there are as many different views of what research is as there are writers who offer such views. We have attempted to synthesize these views and offer the following description of what research is:

> Research is a scientific process of inquiry and/or experimentation that involves purposeful, systematic and rigorous collection of data. Analysis and interpretation of

the data are then made in order to gain new knowledge or add to existing knowledge. Research has the ultimate aim of developing an organized body of scientific knowledge.

What Research Is Not

Before we look further at the explanation of what research *is*, let us take some time to look at what research *is not*. Research is not going to the library to collect existing information on a specific topic, then writing a review of the material such as a "term paper" or "research project." This activity involves the reorganization and/or restatement of already known knowledge and is sometimes referred to as a "search" rather than research. In order to be considered scientific research, present and past knowledge must be used to answer *new* questions, and to add *new* knowledge to the fund of already existing knowledge. Research activity is intended to find answers to questions or solutions for problems. Communicating knowledge that already exists, therefore, is not considered research activity unless new questions are answered or new problems solved. Research is conducted only after an extensive examination of materials related to the proposed question or problem has been carried out. This examination determines if the answer to the question or problem is available in present knowledge. If correct answers are readily available, there is no need for new research unless the researcher suspects an error or seeks an alternative solution.

Now that we have taken a look at some of the things research is not, let's return to our previous description of what research is. Again, research can be described as a scientific process of inquiry and/or experimentation that involves purposeful, systematic and rigorous collection of data. Analysis and interpretation of the data are then made, in order to gain new knowledge or add to existing knowledge, with the ultimate aim of developing an organized body of scientific knowledge.

Research as a Scientific Process of Inquiry

Science is a branch of knowledge or study concerned with deriving systematized knowledge by establishing and organizing facts, principles and methods. The goal of science is developing theories to explain, predict, and/or control phenomena.

The Scientific Method

In research, the scientific method is utilized. This method is an orderly process that utilizes the principles of science; it requires the use of certain sequential steps to acquire dependable information in solving problems. The scientific method is characterized by: (1) order; (2) control; (3) empiricism; (4) generalization and theoretical formulation.[1]

Order

The scientific approach to problem solving requires that order and discipline be applied so that confidence in the investigation's results can be assured. This entails the use of the scientific method in which a series of systematic steps is followed: identification of a problem to be investigated, collection of information according to a previously designed plan (which bears on the solution of the problem), analysis of the information, and formulation of conclusions regarding the problem being investigated.

Control

Control of factors not relevant to the investigation is an essential element of the scientific method. This means that the investigator must attempt to identify the effects of factors *not* being directly investigated in connection with the identi-

---

1. Denise Polit and Bernadette Hungler. *Nursing Research: Principles and Methods* (Philadelphia: J. B. Lippincott, 1978), pp. 20–22.

fied problem, and attempt to keep them from influencing those factors identified for study. For example, in investigating the relationship between cerebrovascular accidents and the Pill, the investigator must take measures to control such influences as stress, diet, and other factors contributing to the development of atherosclerosis.

Empiricism

The scientific method is also characterized by empiricism. That is, the evidence gathered to generate new knowledge must be rooted in objective reality, and be gathered directly or indirectly through the human senses.

Generalization

Generalization, which is one characteristic of the scientific method, means that the investigator does not utilize the scientific method merely to understand isolated events, but must also be able to apply the investigation's results to a broader setting. The ultimate aim of a study that investigated the effects of applying topical insulin to patients with decubitus ulcers (Appendix A) was not limited to an analysis of the effects of topical insulin on the patients in the study. It was designed to draw conclusions regarding the effect of the treatment on ulcer patients in general. The kinds of generalizations that result from such research studies assist in the development of scientific theories, thus providing explanations and predictions of future events.

Purposes of Research

Research involves finding answers to questions or solutions to problems, the discovery and interpretation of new facts, the testing of theories in order to revise accepted theories and/or laws in the light of new facts, and the formulation of new theories. Finally, research has as its ultimate aim the development of an organized body of scientific knowledge that is systematized and that can be useful in explaining, predicting and/or controlling phenomena.

Research in Nursing

Nursing research, then, is research conducted to answer questions or find solutions to specific nursing problems. This is done to develop an organized body of scientific knowledge which is unique to nursing:

> Research in nursing investigates the area of knowledge where the physical and behavioral sciences meet and influence one another, in an effort to study how health problems relate to human behavior and how behavior relates to health and illness.[2]

The goal of nursing research is to improve the practice and profession of nursing for the ultimate improvement of patient care.

Limitations of the Scientific Research Process

Although the scientific research process is usually considered the highest form of attaining human knowledge, it has a number of limitations involving the types of problems that can be investigated. Questions involving morality or value systems cannot be explored with the scientific research approach; questions dealing with complex social and psychological phenomena—such as anger and anxiety—are also very difficult to investigate because of the problems involved in measuring these phenomena. When human subjects need to be used in the study, constraints to protect them often cause additional difficulties. Such constraints have even precluded the application of the scientific method to the investigation of certain problems. This is a very crucial consideration and is discussed in greater detail in later chapters.

---

2. *Research in Nursing* (Kansas City: American Nurses' Association, 1976), p. 1.

Classification of Research Activities

It will be helpful to know the meaning of some commonly used research terms utilized to classify research activities if you are going to understand research.

Classification By Purpose

Research may be classified by *purpose,* that is, *basic research* or *applied research.* This classification reflects the degree to which the findings can be applied to practical problems in the every day world. *Basic research,* also called pure research, is concerned with establishing new knowledge and with the development or refinement of theories. The findings of basic research may not be immediately applicable to practical problems, but they do provide basic scientific knowledge for building further research. Basic research is really "knowledge for the sake of knowledge." This is in contrast to *applied research* which is also concerned with establishing new knowledge, but is further concerned that the knowledge can be applied in practical settings without undue delay. Applied research has been referred to as practical application of the theoretical. In general, basic research in the behavioral sciences serves to discover general laws concerning human behavior, while applied research generates knowledge about the operation of these laws in specific settings. However, the distinction between basic and applied research often may not be as clear cut as we have described. Sometimes the results of basic research studies can be applied in a practical setting, while findings from applied research studies can serve as the focus for basic research.

The majority of nursing studies are instances of applied research. For example, the studies conducted by Lindeman on the value of structured preoperative teaching, deep breathing, coughing, and bed exercises have immediate application in practical settings.[3] There have been some basic research

---

3. Carol A. Lindeman and Betty Van Aernam, "Nursing Intervention With the Presurgical Patient—The Effects of Structured and

studies conducted in nursing, such as McKinnon-Mullett's study concerned with circulation research and its potential in clinical nursing research.[4]

Classification by Approach

Research may also be classified by *approach*. There are three major approaches: *descriptive, experimental,* and *historical.* In the *descriptive research approach,* questions are based on the ongoing events of the present which describe what exists now. In the *experimental research approach,* questions are based on the necessity of manipulating specific conditions in a controlled or laboratory-like setting in order to investigate the effects of different conditions. In the *historical research approach,* questions based on the past are investigated by utilizing procedures to determine the accuracy of statements or facts about past events. Each of these approaches is discussed in more detail in the chapters in Part 3.

Why Should Nurses Learn About Research?

One of the characteristics of a professional group is that it has a unique body of knowledge and skill. It is generally agreed that nursing is still in the process of defining not only what nursing is, but also what constitutes its unique body of knowledge and skill. In view of this, nursing needs to direct its efforts toward systematic investigation of questions related to the practice and profession of nursing.

Unstructured Preoperative Teaching." *Nursing Research,* 20 (July–August 1971):319–332; Carol A. Lindeman, "Nursing Intervention with the Presurgical Patient: Effectiveness and Efficiency of Group and Individual Preoperative Teaching—Phase Two." *Nursing Research,* 21 (May–June 1972):196–209.

4. Elizabeth McKinnon-Mullett, "Approaches to the Study of Nursing Questions and the Development of Nursing Science. Circulation Research: Exploring Its Potential in Clinical Nursing Research," *Nursing Research,* 21 (November–December 1972):494–498.

In the 1976 Guidelines prepared by the Commission on Nursing Research of the American Nurses' Association, the essential nature of research in improving nursing practice was recognized:

> This points to the need for greater emphasis on education for research for the improvement of practice. . . . As more nurses are prepared for participation in research through undergraduate, graduate, and continuing education, new knowledge resulting from research should increasingly pertain to the effects of nursing intervention and care, and an observable impact on practice can be expected.[5]

The guidelines also define elements of competence in research that are "essential to the development of sound researchers and practitioners" and should be integrated throughout the nursing educational process.

If nursing is to develop an organized body of scientific knowledge, there are several ways in which you as a nurse can contribute. First, you must become a sophisticated consumer of the results of research conducted by others. You need to be able to evaluate the studies' contributions to scientific knowledge so that you can decide whether or not to utilize this knowledge in the care of your patients. The material in Chapter 6 will provide you with principles and techniques to guide you in this evaluation process. With a basic research orientation, you will also be able to generate hunches and raise questions on which research studies can be carried out. Finally, you may want to become involved in a research project that will contribute to new knowledge, either as a principal investigator or as a participant.

Although the emphasis on research in nursing has become a relatively strong movement only within the past twenty years, historically nursing research has been emerging over a period of one hundred years. The next section pro-

---

5. *Preparation of Nurses for Participation in Research* (Kansas City: American Nurses' Association, 1976).

vides a brief overview of the historical development of aspects of nursing which have significantly affected the development of nursing research.

Nursing Research Over the Years

When Florence Nightingale established her system of nursing and nursing education over one hundred years ago, she envisioned the development of a scholarly, humane, and scientific discipline. She utilized the research approach to observe situations and used her detailed records to formulate ideas on ways to improve nursing and health care. She encouraged nurses to develop the habit of sound observation:

> In dwelling upon the vital importance of *sound* observation, it must never be lost sight of what observation is for. It is not for the sake of piling up miscellaneous information or curious facts, but for the sake of saving life and increasing health and comfort.[6]

If nursing education in the United States had followed the principles to which Florence Nightingale was dedicated, nursing research might have progressed more swiftly. However, the development of hospital schools of nursing, with their primary emphasis on nursing service by students, resulted in nurses being placed in subservient roles. They cared primarily for ill persons and meticulously carried out the orders of authority figures, usually physicians. Unfortunately for the progress of nursing research, nurses who accepted these subservient roles were hardly able to develop or refine the questioning attitude and abstract thinking associated with the scientific method of inquiry.

From 1900 to 1950, the majority of leaders in nursing had advanced preparation in the field of education. This resulted in many of the research studies conducted centering around education for nursing rather than the practice of nursing. The majority of these research studies were con-

---

6. Florence Nightingale, *Notes on Nursing* (Philadelphia: J. B. Lippincott, 1859), p. 70.

cerned with the characteristics of nursing students themselves, as well as their educational preparation.

Articles in the nursing literature from 1900 to 1950 show nurses concerned and writing about the care of patients with communicable diseases, hygiene and sanitation, asepsis, and high maternal and infant death rates. The first case studies appeared in the *American Journal of Nursing* during the 1920s and were used as teaching tools for students, as well as patient progress records to improve patient care. By 1930, the need to distinguish nursing orders from medical orders and to evaluate the effectiveness of nursing procedures appeared. Articles began to express the need for student nurses to be free to criticize, and to be relieved of excessive nursing service duties in order to benefit fully from their educational programs.

In the late 1940s, following World War II, the broader concept of nursing as practiced by public health nurses became accepted. The primary focus on nursing care for the hospitalized patient was expanded to include the patient and family in a variety of settings, in cooperation with physicians and other health professionals, and the prevention of illness and the promotion of health. An awareness grew of the need for nurses to acquire knowledge of the social, behavioral, and natural sciences, and the humanities, in order to utilize this knowledge in caring for their patients and families.

In the 1950s, recognition of the need to prepare nurses at the graduate level for leadership positions, advanced practice, and research contributed to the advancement of nursing research.

In order to communicate the growing body of nursing research, the first issue of *Nursing Research* was published in 1952. This journal serves as an important resource devoted to issues and problems associated with nursing research and to the publication of nursing research studies. In 1955, the American Nurses' Association established the American Nurses' Foundation, which supports and promotes research in nursing, and furthers the dissemination of research findings.

Nurses writing since the 1950s have reflected ideas about

the conceptual development of nursing, nursing as a science, and the educational preparation needed for nurses to conduct research.

From 1955 to 1965 was again an important time for research related to nursing education. Researchers focused on student characteristics, selection and retention of students, as well as the educational process. Articles dealing with the quality of patient care began to appear in the literature. Research studies focused on long-term care and rehabilitation of patients and on problems of patients with chronic diseases such as heart disease, cancer, and stroke. Hospitals began to report experiences with intensive care units and automation.

In 1970, the National Commission for the Study of Nursing and Nursing Education reported that little research had been done on the actual effects of nursing intervention and care and that nursing had few definitive guides for the improvement of practice:

> Lack of research leaves us without a body of facts or a set of probabilities to guide or assess the nursing care of a patient. Of necessity, nursing practice today consists of stereotyped techniques sprinkled liberally with personal idiosyncrasy. . . . Since we have not developed valid means for assessing the effects of varied interventions, it is almost impossible to define optimum nursing care.[7]

The 1973 report [8] emphasized that nursing today is still more of an art than a science. Nurse–patient interactions are characterized by a combination of individual judgment, concern for the patient, and supportive care rather than with procedures based on validated scientific knowledge. However, with the increased amount and complexity of knowl-

---

7. National Commission for the Study of Nursing and Nursing Education, *An Abstract for Action* (New York: McGraw-Hill, 1970), p. 84.
8. National Commission for the Study of Nursing and Nursing Education, *From Abstract into Action* (New York: McGraw-Hill, 1973), p. 125.

edge concerning human health and response to illness, the art of nursing is no longer sufficient to assure optimum patient care. Continued scientific and systematic investigation is needed to elevate the practice of nursing to both an art and a science.

In 1976, the American Nurses' Association developed a statement of priorities for research in nursing. These priorities were designed to guide nurse researchers in the study of areas of nursing which are crucial to the advancement of the nursing profession. They fall into two major areas: (1) questions related to the practice of nursing and (2) questions related to the profession of nursing.[9]

Currently, there have been major expansions in research related to clinical practice, increasing concerns with ethical practices, and the protection of human subjects. Nurses are increasingly studying *nursing*—they see an urgent need to investigate the organization and delivery of nursing care to patients. Future trends in nursing research indicate an increased concentration on research designed to investigate existing nursing practice and to develop theories that will guide nursing practice. The ultimate goal is to extend the scientific knowledge base for nursing practice in order to improve patient care.

In this chapter we introduced you to some of the basic concepts related to research and nursing research, as well as providing a brief overview of the historical development of the nursing research movement in the United States.

The following application activities should help you apply this information.

Application Activities

1. Formulate your own definition of nursing research which encompasses the concepts found in the various definitions in the literature.

---

9. *Priorities for Research in Nursing* (Kansas City: American Nurses' Association, 1976).

2. Read the research study reprinted in Appendix A. Using the definition of research presented in the chapter, discuss how the study fulfills the definition:

   a. The study is a scientific process of inquiry and/or experimentation.

   b. The study involves systematic and rigorous collection of data.

   c. The study involves analysis and interpretation of data.

   d. The study was designed to gain new knowledge which has the potential to contribute to an organized body of scientific knowledge.

   e. How could this study contribute to improved nursing practice for better patient care?

   f. Classify the study by research purpose: is it basic or applied research? Why?

   g. Classify the study by research approach: is it survey, experimental, or historical research? Why?

3. It has been stated that nurses should conduct their own research into the practice and profession of nursing. Do you agree or disagree with this statement? Defend your answer.

Bibliography and Suggested Readings

American Nurses' Association. *Preparation of Nurses For Participation In Research.* Code No. D–54 2500. Kansas City: The Association, 1976.

———. *Priorities for Research in Nursing.* Code No. D–51 3M. Kansas City: The Association, August 1976.

———. *Research in Nursing.* Kansas City: The Association, 1976.

Gortner, Susan and Nahm, Helen. "An Overview of Nursing Research in the United States," *Nursing Research,* 26 (January–February 1977): 10–30.

Hopkins, Charles D. *Educational Research: A Structure for Inquiry.* Columbus: Charles E. Merrill Publishing Co., 1976.

Lindeman, Carol A. "Nursing Intervention With the Presurgical Patient: Effectiveness and Efficiency of Group and Individual Preoperative Teaching—Phase Two," *Nursing Research,* 21 (May–June 1972): 196–209.

————. "Nursing Research: A Visible, Viable Component of Nursing Practice," *Journal of Nursing Administration,* Vol. III (March–April 1973): 18–21.

———— and Van Aernam, Betty. "Nursing Intervention With the Presurgical Patient—The Effects of Structured and Unstructured Preoperative Teaching," *Nursing Research,* 20 (July–August 1971): 319–332.

McKinnon-Mullett, Elizabeth. "Approaches to the Study of Nursing Questions and the Development of Nursing Science. Circulation Research: Exploring its Potential in Clinical Nursing Research," *Nursing Research,* 21 (November–December 1972): 494–498.

National Commission for the Study of Nursing and Nursing Education. *An Abstract For Action.* New York: McGraw-Hill, 1970.

————. *From Abstract into Action.* New York: McGraw-Hill, 1973.

National League for Nursing. *Theory Development: What, Why, How?* New York: N.L.N. Publication, Code No. 15-1708, 1978.

Nightingale, Florence. *Notes on Nursing.* Philadelphia: J. B. Lippincott, 1859.

Polit, Denise and Hungler, Bernadette. *Nursing Research: Principles and Methods.* Philadelphia: J. B. Lippincott, 1978.

Part 2

Applying the Research Process to Nursing Problems

The material in Part 2 is designed to acquaint you with the stages of the research process; it also presents principles and activities for applying the research process to nursing problems.

Chapter 2 presents an overview of the stages of the research process. Chapter 3 focuses on the selection and statement of the research problem, including review of related literature, formulation of a conceptual of theoretical framework, and purpose for the study.

Chapter 4 presents a discussion of data collection principles and techniques. Chapter 5 discusses data analysis. Chapter 6 focuses on the final stage of the research process—communicating the research results.

2

Stages of the Research Process

THIS chapter is designed to acquaint you with the nature of the research process and its relationship to the problem solving process. It describes the three stages of the research process that are utilized in conducting a research study.

Overview of the Research Process

As you become acquainted with research terminology, you will see the term *research process* used to refer to the systematic steps, or ongoing phases, involved in conducting a research study. While the number and order of these steps may vary, the following outline contains those commonly used:

1. Statement of the research problem
2. Review of related literature
3. Statement of the purpose of the study
4. Collection of data
5. Analysis and interpretation of data
6. Formulation of conclusions and implications
7. Communication of the results of the study

Remember, conducting a study using the research process is a systematic, planned activity that can be thought of as a chain of reasoning. It begins with a statement of the problem and systematically proceeds through to communication of the study's results. "The total process from problem isolation to the addition of new knowledge is a logically structured inquiry into some well-defined problem." [1]

Relationship of the Research Process to the Problem Solving Process

Even though research and problem solving are often compared, it is important to understand that the research process and the problem solving process are not the same. Basically, the two differ in purpose. Problem solving is simpler than the research process; its purpose is to find an immediate solution to a practical problem in an actual setting. The basic purpose of research, on the other hand, goes beyond solving the immediate problem; it provides new knowledge that can be generalized to a broader setting and benefit large numbers of people. For example, the nurse may decide that the application of topical insulin to a patient's decubitus ulcer is an effective solution to a particular patient care problem. In contrast, a systematic research study (such as the study reprinted in Appendix A), conducted in relation to the same patient care problem of decubitus ulcers, would be expected to benefit a large number of patients.

Comparison between Research and Problem Solving

Table 2–1 compares research and problem solving and summarizes the elements essential to research, and describes the differences of parallel elements to problem solving. Placing the research problem within the context of existing knowledge, as well as within a theoretical or conceptual framework, is an additional element of research. Problem solving does not include this requirement.

---

1. Charles D. Hopkins. *Educational Research: A Structure for Inquiry* (Columbus: Charles E. Merrill Publishing Co., 1976), p. 13.

Table 2-1

ELEMENTS OF RESEARCH AND PROBLEM SOLVING *

RESEARCH	PROBLEM SOLVING
All elements of a scientific inquiry must be explicitly and precisely described.	The same explicitness and precision, though they may be utilized, are not usually demanded of problem solving.
Where research data are quantitative or quantifiable, they are analyzed with appropriate statistical procedures.	Detailed statistical analyses are seldom done, and quantitative data are usually limited to simple frequency counts.
Elaborate pains are taken to control for factors other than the variable under study.	Such controls are not imposed.
A primary aim is to ensure that findings are generalizable to a population larger than the one subject to study.	The primary aim is the solution of a problem existing in the population being studied; addresses little or no attention to whether findings may be expected to apply to a larger population.

---

* Mabel Wandelt. *Guide for the Beginning Researcher* (New York: Appleton-Century-Crofts, 1970), pp. xvii–xviii. Used with permission of Appleton-Century-Crofts.

Which Approach Is "Better"?

Once you understand that the research process and the problem solving process have different purposes, it follows that the use of one process rather than the other to investigate a problem should not be considered more valuable or better. The value lies in correctly utilizing the process most appropriate for the investigation.

Table 2–1 (continued)

RESEARCH	PROBLEM SOLVING
The search for new knowledge through hypothesis testing must be done in a setting and with study subjects different from those which gave rise to the observations that prompted the study and hypotheses (lest there be circularity: from problem, to evidence, to "proof").	The facts for the investigation are always gathered in the same setting and from many of the same subjects that gave rise to the proposal that the study be done.
Entails a plan written in sufficient detail and explicitness that the study may be replicated and the findings verified.	Entails no such requirements.
The researcher has the moral obligation to report his findings in writing that others may share the new knowledge.	The problem solver needs only to provide information, in verbal or tabular form, to those in the immediate setting of the problem and to propose changes that will help them solve the problem that prompted the study.

Stages of the Research Process

It is helpful to consider the research process as consisting of three sequential stages that are designed to answer the research question or to solve the research problem: (1) the planning stage, (2) the implementation stage, (3) the communication stage.

Stage I: Planning the Study

The initial stage of the research process is the planning stage. Here the problem question, which the research will answer, is selected and refined into a problem statement, and the methodology for the study is formulated. The problem must be researchable and the answer not already known. The research should contribute to new knowledge. Appropriate methods must be available to investigate the problem. Consideration must be given to the availability of subjects expected to participate in the study, as well as the research's ethical implications, such as the protection of the study participants' rights. The constraints of time and money imposed by the study are also important considerations in selecting the problem for the research study. To place the problem in the context of what is already known, the researcher then reviews the literature related to the problem, citing references to significant publications and journal articles that pertain to the problem. Since the objective of nursing research is to contribute to scientific knowledge, the problem may be placed within a theory or based upon concepts to which the study's results can be related. The literature review summarizes existing knowledge in relation to work done on the problem, as well as assisting the investigator in learning more about the problem area. Next in the planning stage, the researcher may use the information gained so far to predict the outcome of the study. This is done by formulating a hypothesis—an educated guess—that will be used to guide the rest of the study. The testing of the hypothesis then becomes the purpose for conducting the study. Not all research studies are conducted to test hypotheses; some studies are designed to answer questions or to describe phenomena.

All of the terms relating to the study must be carefully defined so there will be no question as to what the researcher means when using the terms.

The methodology for the study defines the way pertinent information will be gathered in order to answer the research question or analyze the research problem. This includes detailed discussion on the selection of subjects who will participate in the study, and description of the data collection procedures and techniques. Also included is a plan for analyzing the data after they have been collected; this assures that they are collected in a form which facilitates analysis. Limitations of the study are included to identify particular aspects of the study over which the researcher has no control.

Thus, the planning stage of the research process consists of the first five steps in the research process: (1) statement of the problem; (2) review of related literature; (3) statement of the purpose of the study; (4) plans for collection of the data; (5) plans for analysis of the data.

In order to structure the planning stage of a research study, the researcher formulates a *research proposal:* a written, detailed description of the proposed study. Sometimes called a prospectus, the research proposal serves as a blueprint for the research project and *must* be completed *prior* to conducting the research study. The written proposal communicates the problem being investigated and the procedures that will be used in the investigation. A research proposal is written for several purposes. The process of having to sit down and write a proposal for the research study forces the researcher to think through the various aspects of the study which might not otherwise have been considered. The plan can then be evaluated by others who may help to improve it by suggesting something that has been left out, and whether or not the ideas would be workable in the actual study setting. The written proposal provides a step-by-step guide to follow in carrying out the research project; it saves having to remember the many details already considered and the anticipated problems already solved. A well thought out proposal saves time, helps avoid mistakes, and should result in a higher quality research study.

Written research proposals are required for all academic research studies, such as theses and dissertations, and for all research submitted for funding by various governmental agencies and private organizations. Although you are

not now in a position to develop such a sophisticated proposal, writing your own proposal will help you to learn more
about the research process by actually applying it to a nursing problem of your own choice. Remember, research is
a learned activity. All those who are now capable of writing
sophisticated research proposals were once beginning research students like yourselves.

In developing a research proposal (Stage I of the planning stage of the research process), information related to
the first five steps of the research process is included; it is
generally agreed that the following information should be
included in a research proposal. Each of these components
will be discussed in more detail in subsequent chapters.
Step-by-step guidelines for the development of a research
proposal are included in Appendix G.

1. Statement of the problem
   This section should include the background of the problem
   as well as a brief statement of what is being investigated.
   The significance of the study should also be stated.
2. Review of related literature
   This section presents summaries of other studies and articles
   that are related to the problem. It may also include the
   concepts or theory on which the research is based.
3. Statement of the purpose of the study
   This section contains a clear statement of the purpose for
   conducting the research. It may be stated as a hypothesis to
   be tested, a question to be answered, or phenomenon to be
   described or analyzed.
4. Definitions of the terms used in the study
5. Plan for data collection
   This section should include detailed descriptions of the
   study subjects selected, and should describe the data collection techniques and procedures. Assumptions and limitations of the study may be included here.
6. Plan for data analysis
   This section contains procedures for analyzing the study
   data, including the kinds of tables to be used. If you plan

to carry out a study, but do not have a statistical background, you will need to get help with this section of your proposal.

7. Bibliography
8. Appendices (optional)

   This section may include materials developed especially for the study (cover letters, consent forms, questionnaires, interview schedules, and so forth).

Stage II: Implementing the Research Proposal

After the completed research proposal has been evaluated by those who can offer suggestions, and perhaps has been revised to incorporate their suggestions, it must be approved by the appropriate institutional committees. This is very important, for it assures the protection of the rights of the study subjects as well as conformity to the policies and procedures of the institution. The researcher is then ready to implement the written proposal. The implementation stage of the research process is where the actual collection and analysis of data for the research study takes place. In this stage, the researcher follows the written proposal by systematically gathering the data for analysis. If unexpected problems arise in the research situation, the researcher may decide to alter the procedures while still implementing the written proposal as closely as possible.

Stage III: Communicating the Results of the Study

After analyzing the data in relation to the research problem, the researcher formulates and discusses conclusions, and relates these conclusions to relevant present knowledge. The researcher should cite implications of the research and formulate recommendations for further study. The researcher then writes a report of the complete study to communicate its findings so that others have access to the knowledge. Research reports vary from formal reports to abridged reports for publication. A formal research report usually contains the following information and will be discussed further in Chapter 6.

The research report is divided into three major parts: preliminary materials, main body (text) of the report, and reference materials. Each main part consists of several sections:

1. Preliminary materials

   This section includes the title page, table of contents, list of illustrations or figures, list of tables, and a preface or acknowledgment, if any.

2. Main body (text) of the report

   A. *The introduction section* includes the statement of the problem, review of related literature, conceptual or theoretical framework, purpose of the study, and definition of terms.

   B. *The methodology section* includes the research approach, a description of the study subjects, techniques for data collection, procedures, assumptions and limitations of the study.

   C. *The findings section* includes the presentation of the data that have been collected for the study.

   D. *The discussion section* includes interpretation of findings by the investigator, implications for nursing, and recommendations for further study.

   E. *The summary section* includes a brief restatement of the problem, purpose, major findings, conclusions and recommendations.

3. Reference materials

   This section includes the bibliography and appendices.

Comparing these components of the research report with those of a research proposal, you will see that the completed research report has the added components of data analysis and interpretation, as well as conclusions and recommendations for further study. This is logical when you recall that the proposal is written in the planning stage of the research process and describes what the researcher purports to do. The completed research report represents the implementation stage and describes what the researcher actually did and found.

The research proposal is written in the future tense; much of it may be utilized in writing the research report by changing it to the past tense.

In this chapter, we considered the nature and components of the research process and its relation to the problem solving process. The research process was presented as three sequential stages: *The planning stage* in which a research proposal is written to describe the study problem and methodology; *The implementation stage* in which the completed research proposal is implemented to collect and analyze the data; *The communication stage* in which the researcher formulates conclusions and implications for the study, and writes up the report of the study in order to communicate the new knowledge. In order to apply the principles presented, you should complete the application activities listed below.

Application Activities

1. Choose a published nursing research study and use the comparison of the elements of research and problem solving presented in the chapter to:
   a. *Systematically* analyze the investigator's use of the research process rather than the problem solving process.
   b. Is the study applied or basic research? Why?
   c. Is the study descriptive, historical or experimental research? Why?
2. Read the research proposal in Appendix D which was written by a beginning researcher. This proposal represents the planning stage of the research process and should help you understand the type of information a research proposal contains and what a completed proposal looks like. This researcher planned to implement her proposal and received help from her instructors with the data analysis section of the proposal. You may also want to read the research proposals in Appen-

dices B and C which were also written by beginning research students. They represent the historical research approach and the descriptive research approach, respectively. These students also received help in writing the data analysis sections of their proposals.

3. The student who wrote the research proposal in Appendix D was able to implement her proposal and conduct the study. Reading her research report in Appendix E should help you understand the relationship between a research proposal and a completed research report. Notice how the research proposal is used in the research report by changing it to the past tense. As a beginning researcher, this student also received help in writing the data analysis section of her report.

Bibliography and Suggested Readings

Brink, Pamela J. and Wood, Marilynn. *Basic Steps in Planning Nursing Research*. North Scituate: Duxbury Press, 1978.

Fox, David J. *Fundamentals of Research in Nursing*. 3rd ed. New York: Appleton-Century-Crofts, 1976.

Hopkins, Charles D. *Educational Research: A Structure For Inquiry*. Columbus: Charles E. Merrill Publishing Co., 1976.

Polit, Denise and Hungler, Bernadette. *Nursing Research: Principles and Methods*. Philadelphia: J. B. Lippincott Co., 1978.

Van Dalen, Deobold B. *Understanding Educational Research*. New York: McGraw Hill Book Co., 1973.

Wandelt, Mabel. *Guide For the Beginning Researcher*. New York: Appleton-Century-Crofts, 1970.

3

Problem Selection and Statement

I n Chapter 2, the research process was described as a chain of reasoning that begins with a statement of the problem and systematically proceeds through to communication of the study's results.

The material in this chapter is designed to acquaint you with the initial step of the research process: selection and statement of the research problem. This is an extremely important component in the research process. It begins with the identification of a general problem area of interest and involves the subsequent narrowing down of the topic to a very specific problem to be investigated. Although the researcher is not expected to identify a research problem until after doing some relevant reading, it is important to become familiar with the sources of research problems and with the criteria for evaluating them.

Selection of a Researchable Problem

The selection of the problem to be investigated is an extremely important step and determines to a large extent the nature and quality of the research. Think of the problem as a question needing to be answered or as a situation needing a solution. First, look at your professional experiences and describe a situation that aroused your interest—even one that annoyed you—and led you to think that something ought to be done about this or that surely it could be done a better way. Examples of general problem areas in nursing might include preoperative teaching for mastectomy patients, discharge planning for premature infants, successful breast feeding in primiparas, or medication errors made by post-hospitalized geriatric patients. If you find that your own experience fails to generate a problem area, use the library for locating literature related to your area of professional interest.

Having identified a general problem area related to your particular area of interest and experience, narrow it down to one specific problem which is manageable within the research process. A problem which is too broad will cause difficulties. It can result in a study that will be too general, or too difficult to conduct and interpret the results. It is often helpful to state the problem as a question. For example, the general problem area of successful breast feeding in primiparas could be narrowed down by asking the question, "What is the effect of teaching about breast feeding to primiparas?" This might then generate such problems as "What are the differences in comparable success with breast feeding in primiparas taught specific concepts and techniques related to breast feeding versus primiparas not exposed to such teaching?" or "What is the effect of individualized versus group instruction on successful breast feeding practices in primiparas?"

It is well worth the time and effort it takes to select a worthwhile problem specific enough to result in a manageable study. In your efforts to narrow down a general problem area, however, be careful not to go to the point where it becomes so trivial that it is not worth the time and the effort involved in researching it.

Sources of Research Problems

There are several major sources of problems that need to be researched. An obvious source is the researcher's own background and personal experiences. As a nurse, you are in an excellent position to identify researchable problems unique to nursing. Another important source of research-able topics is the literature. Research studies reported in various nursing and related journals provide many kinds of problems observed by other researchers. Many studies raise additional questions, or include recommendations for further study, that can form the basis of new studies. A study that has already been conducted can be replicated in a different setting to see if its findings can be generalized.

A third source of research problems is theory. Investigation of problems derived from theory provides the most meaningful contribution to scientific knowledge. A theory is not merely a body of facts, it provides an explanation of facts which are used as principles to explain or predict certain phenomenon. A good theory can guide research by pointing to areas that need to be investigated, and research can contribute to the related theory by confirming or failing to confirm some aspect of the theory:

> The more research is directed by scientific theory, the more likely are its results to contribute directly to the development and further organization of a scientific body of knowledge in nursing.[1]

Beginning researchers may find the selection of a problem based on theory too sophisticated at this stage of their education. However, it is necessary to be aware of this source of research problems, and the importance of designing nursing research studies that contribute to nursing's scientific knowledge base.

Problem Selection Criteria

There are certain major characteristics of a well selected research problem that should be considered. A researcher should evaluate a proposed problem and decide if it should be pursued through the research process by asking the following questions:

---

1. Faye Abdellah and Eugene Levine, *Better Patient Care through Nursing Research* (2nd ed.), New York: The Macmillan Co., 1979, p. 75.

1. Is the topic of interest?
2. Is it "researchable"?
3. Is it practicable?
4. Is it significant?
5. Is it ethical to conduct research on this problem?

Is the Topic Interesting?

Since the researcher will become deeply involved in planning and implementing the research study, the topic should be one which will sustain interest over a prolonged period of time.

Is the Problem Researchable?

A researchable problem is one that can be investigated through the collection and analysis of data which exist in the real world. The meanings of the concepts must be clear and you must be able to present them through tangible, observable evidence; that is, evidence obtained through direct observation or through other activities that will provide similar evidence relating to the concept.

Is the Problem Practicable?

A research problem is practicable if it is possible to carry out the necessary related activities. Even if the topic is of interest to you, and in your area of expertise, you will need to consider the following: are appropriate methodology and resources available in terms of suitable measuring instruments or equipment? are subjects available? and will you have cooperation from others? You also need to consider the length of time needed to complete the study as well as the cost involved.

Is the Problem Significant?

Even though your topic may be interesting itself, you need to consider if it is sufficiently significant to warrant a study. A good nursing research problem has either practical or theoretical significance; its solution contributes to the improvement of nursing care or to the advancement of nursing as a profession by providing scientific knowledge or theoretical formulations.

In 1976, the American Nurses' Association Committee on Nursing Research developed a list of priorities to serve as guidelines for the study of areas crucial to the improvement of nursing practice and to the advancement of nursing as a profession. The priorities fall into two areas:

1. Questions related to the practice of nursing and
2. Questions related to the profession of nursing.

Examples of priorities in the practice area include: (1) Studies to reduce complications of hospitalization and surgery (sleep deprivation, anorexia, diarrhea, neurosensory disturbances, respiratory infections, circulatory problems, and others); (2) Studies to improve the outlook for high risk parents and high risk infants; (3) Studies to improve the health care of the elderly. Examples of priorities in the profession area include: (1) Studies of manpower for nursing education, practice, and research; (2) Studies of quality assurance for nursing and studies of criterion measures for practice and education.[2]

The twelve practice areas priorities and the six profession areas priorities are further described in an article by de Tornyay and may assist you in choosing a significant research problem.[3]

Is the Research Ethical?

Finally, you must evaluate the ethical implications of your problem to protect the rights of the subjects who would participate in the study. Obtaining informed consent from participants, protecting them from harm, and maintaining

2. American Nurses' Association, *Priorities for Research in Nursing,* Code No. D-51 3M (Kansas City: The Association, May, 1976).
3. Rheba de Tornyay, "Nursing Research—The Road Ahead," *Nursing Research* 26 (November–December 1977):404–407.

anonymity and confidentiality are major considerations. The 1968 guidelines for the nurse in research approved by the American Nurses' Association Board of Directors include specific statements regarding: (1) the nurse in the research setting; (2) protection of human rights; (3) manner of consent; (4) drugs used in research; and (5) animals in research.[4]

The 1975 *Human Rights Guidelines for Nurses in Clinical and Other Research* updated the earlier statement and was accepted by the Commission on Nursing Research of the American Nurses' Association. This position statement on human rights for nurses engaged in research activity is intended to reflect the immense social and technological changes that profoundly affect the scope of nursing responsibility. Guidelines are included for: (1) the types of activities involved in the protection of human rights; (2) the rights that are to be protected; (3) the persons to be safeguarded; and (4) mechanisms necessary to ensure that protection is adequate.[5] This extremely important area on the protection of human rights is discussed further in Appendix F and will help you evaluate the ethical aspects of your research problem.

In summary, the selection of the research problem—the initial step in the research process—is extremely important and determines the nature and quality of the research study.

Beginning researchers usually need to seek help in evaluating their problem selection, and in deciding if it should be pursued through the research process.

Review of the Related Literature

The initial review of the literature should help you identify and state a research problem. The second review

---

4. American Nurses' Association, "The Nurse in Research: ANA Guidelines on Ethical Values," *American Journal of Nursing* 68 (July 1968): 1504–1507.

5. American Nurses' Association, *Human Rights Guidelines for Nurses in Clinical and Other Research,* Code No. D-465M (Kansas City: The Association, July, 1975).

involves the systematic identification and analysis of information pertaining to the specific problem you selected for study, and should be done during the initial stages of the research process. Unfortunately, beginning researchers often fail to appreciate the importance of conducting the literature review at this point in the process. In their enthusiasm to proceed with the rest of the study, they fail to put the problem in the perspective of what has already been done.

Why Review the Literature?

There are four primary reasons for conducting a literature review. The first is to determine what has already been done that relates to your problem; this helps avoid the duplication of previous studies and helps you develop a framework for the problem that relates it to completed studies. Since one of the aims of research in nursing is to develop theories of nursing, the literature search may also help you find a theoretical framework within which to investigate the problem. For example, a theory related to learning might form the theoretical framework within which the problem of individual versus group instruction for breast feeding could be investigated. Beginning researchers may not be expected to include a theoretical framework in their studies.

Secondly, the literature review provides ideas on the kinds of studies that need to be done. Previous investigators and writers often make suggestions regarding problems that need further investigation. Reviewing the literature may stimulate the researcher to develop new insights into reported research or to devise new problems to be investigated. Thirdly, the literature review serves to point out research strategies, specific research procedures, and information regarding measuring instruments that have been found productive as well as nonproductive for the problem. Capitalizing on the successes as well as the errors of other researchers helps the researcher to profit from and build upon the experiences of other researchers.

Finally, the literature review can help you interpret the results of the study after it has been conducted by allowing you to discuss the findings in terms of agreement or non-agreement with other studies. Results contradictory to the findings of other studies can suggest further studies to resolve such contradictions.

Recommendations for Locating Pertinent Materials

It is very imortant to become familiar with the available library resources even before beginning the literature review. The time you spend initially in familiarizing yourself with these resources ultimately will save you much valuable time. Try to get a written guide explaining the resources and services of the library and the procedures that need to be followed. It is often helpful to participate in a guided tour of the library so you can learn to utilize the library to its fullest extent. Ask the librarian for help when you need it.

You should become familiar with the use of the card catalogue and locate pertinent encyclopedias and dictionaries, government publications, microfilms and other audiovisual resources. Inquire about interlibrary loans which are designed to assist you in obtaining references not available in your own library. If your library has computerized literature searches such as MEDLARS and MEDLINE, you should investigate them with the librarian to see how they can help you. MEDLARS (*Med*ical *L*iterature *A*nalysis and *R*etrieval *S*ystem) is the computerized literature retrieval service of the National Library of Medicine. MEDLINE is a computerized data base containing approximately 600,000 references to biomedical journal articles published in the United States and 70 foreign countries.

A list of additional computerized literature searches follows; they are valuable sources for locating pertinent references:

AV Line	Audiovisuals-on-line
Bioethics	Ethics, public policy in health care, biomedical research

Cancerlit	Cancer, carcinogenesis, therapy
Cancerproj.	Cancer related grant research projects
Chemline	Chemical dictionary
Clinprot.	Clinical cancer protocols
Epilepsy	Citations on epilepsy
ERIC	Educational Resources Information Center, United States Office of Education
Health	Health care aspects, such as planning
Histline	History of Medicine
PASAR	Psychological Abstracts, American Psychological Association
SOCIOSEARCH	Sociological Abstracts, American Sociological Association
Toxline	Eight abstracting or indexing services on toxicity

Indexes and abstracts are most helpful in identifying relevant references. Indexes are lists of books and articles, or the contents of a book, while abstracts present the main ideas of articles and books. The following indexes and abstracts are the major sources commonly used by nurse researchers:

American Journal of Nursing: Annual and Cumulative Indexes
Biological Abstracts
Bioresearch Index
Child Development Abstracts
Cumulative Index to Nursing Literature

Dissertation Abstracts
Education Index
ERIC
Excerpta Medica
Hospital Literature Index
Index Medicus
International Index
International Nursing Index
Nursing Outlook: Annual and Cumulative Indexes
Nursing Research: Annual and Cumulative Indexes
Nursing Studies Index
Nutrition Abstracts
Psychological Abstracts
Public Health, Social Medicine and Hygiene
Readers' Guide to Periodical Literature
Research Grants Index
Science Citation Index
Sociological Abstracts

In addition to indexes and abstracts, compilations of measuring instruments can be very helpful in identifying relevant references and locating appropriate measuring instruments. The following compilations are specifically related to nursing research:

Ward, Mary Jane and Lindeman, Carol (eds.). *Instruments for Measuring Nursing Practice and Other Care Variables.* 2 vols.; DHEW Publication No. HRA 78–53. Washington: U.S. Government Printing Office, 1978.

Ward, Mary Jane and Fetter, Mark. *Instruments for Use in Nursing Education Research.* Boulder: Western Interstate Commission for Higher Education, 1979.

Following is a list of selected sources for locating measuring instruments that are not specifically related to nursing research, but could relate to your research topic:

Buros, Oscar K. (ed). *Mental Measurements Yearbook.* Highland Park: Gryphon Press, 1975.

Buros, Oscar K. (ed.). *Personality Tests and Reviews.* 2 vols. Highland Park: Gryphon Press, 1970, 1975.

Buros, Oscar K. (ed.). *Tests In Print.* Highland Park: Gryphon Press, 1975.

Chun, KiTaek; Cobb, Sidney; and French, John, Jr. *Measures for Psychological Assessment.* Ann Arbor: University of Michigan Institute for Social Research, 1975.

Goldman, Bert and Saunders, John. *Directory of Unpublished Experimental Measures.* 2 vols.; New York: Behavioral Publications, 1974.

Johnson, Orval. *Tests and Measurements In Child Development: Handbook II.* 2 vols.; San Francisco: Jossey-Bass, Inc., 1976.

Miller, Delbert (ed.). *Handbook of Research Design and Social Measurement.* 2nd ed. New York: McKay, 1970.

Reeder, Leo; Ramacher, Linda; and Gorelnik, S. *Handbook of Scales and Indices of Health Behavior.* Santa Monica, California: Goodyear Publishing Company, 1976.

It is extremely helpful to make a list of key words to guide you in the literature research. For example, key words related to the topic of breast feeding might include nutrition, infant nutrition, newborn, neonatal, nursing, lactation, pregnancy, bottle feeding, mothering, and feminism.

It is preferable to obtain reference material from the primary (original) sources rather than secondary sources; this minimizes error and allows the researcher to analyze the material. Articles you plan to quote directly should be photocopied to reduce citation errors; you should also plan to photocopy all tables and charts cited so that you have the complete information when writing the report.

Of concern to beginning researchers is the amount of time spent on the literature review for writing a research proposal. We concur with Verhonick that, although a hard and fast rule is not easy to state, for a circumscribed study of one semester, two weeks should be appropriate to review literature with the objective of the research kept clearly in mind.[6] The library search application activity at the end of the chapter is designed to assist you in becoming familiar with a large variety of reference sources.

Abstracting the Reference

After locating references which are pertinent to your topic, begin with the latest since this may have additional references from previous research. Read the abstract of the article and/ or the summary to see if the article is pertinent to your topic, then scan the article noting the important points. Plan to use separate index cards (4 × 6 is a convenient size) to record useful information. A separate index card for each reference helps organize the materials when you are ready to write up the literature review. The card should contain the following information:

1. Complete bibliographic reference. Recording this in the format of the style manual required by your department will save you time when you are ready to write the bibliography for your proposal.
2. The complete library call number for a source should be recorded in case you need to recheck it.
3. Developing your own coding system for each reference is useful. Mark such factors as relevance to your study, type of article, and whatever else would be helpful for your research. For example, information concerning the relevance of references could be coded as R+ (very relevant); R (relevant) or R— (less relevant). Information concerning the type of reference could be coded as RS (Research Study) or V (an article expressing the author's viewpoint).
4. Summarize the reference on the card by listing its essential points and noting the important or unusual aspects of the article which will contribute to your study. If you quote di-

---

6. Phyllis Verhonick and Catherine Seamen, *Research Methods for Undergraduate Students in Nursing* (New York: Appleton-Century-Crofts, 1978), p. 24.

rectly from the article, you must copy the quotation word for word, being careful to note that it is a direct quotation.

Writing the Literature Review

After thoroughly investigating the relevant references, you will need to organize them in order to write the literature review if you are preparing a research proposal. You should review the notes on each card in order to refresh your memory, discarding irrelevant references. Include only those references that you used to substantiate your research. Next, make a tentative outline showing the relationships among the topics; then analyze your cards, placing them into the appropriate categories of the outline. For each category, analyze the likenesses and differences between the references. You should summarize references which state essentially the same thing, such as: "Smith (1970), Brown (1974), and Green (1976) report that. . . ." You should include studies which show results contradictory to those you expect to find from your study. When organizing the literature review, discuss the references that are least related to the problem first, logically progressing to the most relevant references. Conclude the review with a brief summary of the main points, general conclusions and implications.

Placing the Problem Within a Theoretical or Conceptual Framework

Beginning researchers are usually unnecessarily frightened or confused by the terms theoretical framework or conceptual framework. Several basic definitions should help. A *concept* is a single idea (often one word) that represents several related component ideas. Examples of concepts are "grief," "alienation," and "happiness." Concepts are the basic ingredients of a *theory* which, in turn, consists of a set of statements called *propositions*. These are stated in such a way as to form a logically interrelated deductive system.

Such a system allows for logically producing new statements from the original set of propositions. A theory can be used to explain and/or predict events (phenomena). Examples of theories include Rotter's social learning theory, Festinger's cognitive dissonance theory, Seyle's adaptation theory, and role theory.

Theoretical Framework

The term theoretical framework merely means the use of one theory or interrelated theories to support the rationale (reason) for conducting the study. For example, Stillman investigated women's health beliefs about breast cancer and breast self-examination within the theoretical framework of cognitive dissonance.[7] Holaday investigated achievement behavior in chronically ill children within the theoretical framework of social learning theory.[8]

Conceptual Framework

The term conceptual framework means the use of two or more concepts to support the rationale for the study problem. When one concept is used, it is the component ideas within it that form the basis for the conceptual framework. The concept may also be discussed in relationship to the variables being investigated in the study. A variable is an observation or measurement that assumes a varying range of values along some dimension. Examples of variables are age, weight, symptoms, ways of behaving.

The student who wrote the research proposal reprinted in Appendix D, investigating the physiologic effects of kinetic nursing in immobilized patients, utilized the conceptual framework of kinetic nursing. The student who

---

7. M. J. Stillman, "Women's Health Beliefs about Breast Cancer and Breast Self-Examination," *Nursing Research,* 26 (March–April 1977):121–127.
8. B. J. Holaday, "Achievement Behavior in Chronically Ill Children," *Nursing Research* 23 (January–February 1974):25–30.

wrote the research proposal reprinted in Appendix C placed her research problem within a theoretical framework using psychoanalytic and adaptation theories.

If nursing research is to make an essential contribution to the scientific knowledge base, each research study should be placed within a theoretical or conceptual framework so that new findings can be placed in the broader areas of already existing knowledge:

> Any one research project provides only a small bit of information, but these bits of information can eventually be brought together to form larger generalizations and conclusions, provided they are all conducted within the same frame of reference and directed toward the same end.[9]

Statement of the Purpose of the Study

The purpose of the study is the single statement that identifies the focus of the research. The purpose should state what you intend to do to answer the research question which generated the problem you are studying. Brink suggests that the statement of the research study's purpose can be written in three ways: 1. as a declarative statement, 2. as a question, or 3. as a hypothesis. The form depends on the way the research question is asked, and the extent of the researcher's knowledge about the problem. The statement of the purpose should include information about the method of collecting the data (such as observe, describe or measure some variable), information about the setting of the study (where you plan to collect the data), and information about the subjects of the study.[10]

---

9. David J. Fox, *Fundamentals of Research in Nursing* (New York: Appleton-Century-Crofts, 1976), p. 28.
10. Pamela J. Brink and Marilyn J. Wood, *Basic Steps in Planning Nursing Research* (North Scituate: Duxbury Press, 1978), pp. 61–62.

The Purpose As a Declarative Statement

In our previously formulated problem designed to describe the relationship between the type of teaching and success in breast feeding by primiparas, the purpose of the study written as a declarative statement could read: "The purpose of this study is to describe the effect of individualized versus group instruction on successful breast feeding by primiparas in their home setting." Note that the statement includes information about the purpose for data collection (to describe), the setting of the study (home setting), and the subjects of the study (primiparas).

The Purpose Stated As a Question

The purpose of the study written as a question could read: "The purpose of this study is to answer the question, What is the effect of individualized versus group instruction on successful breast feeding by primiparas in their home setting?"

The Purpose Stated As a Hypothesis

The purpose of the study written as a hypothesis could read: "The purpose of the study is to test the following hypothesis: Primiparas who receive individualized instruction in breast feeding will have a significantly more successful breast feeding experience in their home setting than primiparas who receive group instruction in breast feeding."

More About Hypotheses

A hypothesis is simply a statement of the predicted relationship between the variables being studied. It is often referred to as the researcher's "educated or calculated guess" as to the study question's answer. It should be supported by existing theory and previous research findings. A study may have more than one hypothesis (which are then referred to as hypotheses). In the statement of a hypothesis, an antecedent condition—called the *independent variable*—is related to the occurrence of another condition or effect called the *dependent variable*. This can be shown as:

Condition X is related to the occurrence of *Condition Y*

Independent variable ——— Dependent variable
(antecedent condition)　　　　　　(effect)

Or

Method of instruction on ——— Degree of success on
breast feeding　　　　　　　breast feeding

    To test the hypothesis, the researcher purposely manipulates the independent variable and attempts to control all the other conditions. The effect on the dependent variable, which occurs presumably as a result of the manipulation of the independent variable, is then noted. Thus, the independent variable comes first in time and is manipulated by the researcher. The dependent variable is the phenomenon that occurs as the researcher alters the independent variable.

Functions of the Hypothesis

Prior to the systematic review of the literature relevant to the research problem, researchers often have a tentative hypothesis, or hypotheses, that express an expectation of the outcome of their study. At this point in the research process, it is necessary to refine and finalize this hypothesis(es), since the hypothesis serves to narrow down the field of the research study and forces the researcher to be precise in stating the specific situation being studied. In addition, the hypothesis guides the methodology for the remainder of the study; that is, the collection of relevant data and the plan for analysis of the data. The hypothesis also serves as a framework for stating conclusions of the study as a direct answer to the hypothesis. A good hypothesis will not only be consistent with theory and previous research, it will also be a reasonable explanation or prediction of the situation being studied. In addition, it will be testable; that is, the researcher will be able to collect data to determine if it can be supported. A hypothesis is not proved, it is either supported or not supported (rejected).

Is a Hypothesis Always Necessary?

A hypothesis can be formulated only if the researcher has enough information to predict the study's outcome and intends to test the significance of the prediction. Although a hypothesis may specify a cause-and-effect relationship, most hypotheses specify a relationship between two or more variables. That is, these variables may exist together, or a change in one will be associated with a change in the other. A hypothesis must be theoretically or conceptually based, and in the case of a cause-and-effect relationship, the base *must* be theory.[11] Thus, a hypothesis is always necessary in an experimental study. It is optional in a descriptive study in which the investigator describes what is, or may use the data to raise questions and/or generate hypotheses for further studies. Many historical research studies have hypotheses that explain the occurrence of events and conditions.

Classification of Hypotheses

You will hear the terms research hypothesis and statistical hypothesis used as classifications. A research hypothesis states the expected relationship between the variables that the researcher expected as the study's outcome. It is stated in the declarative form. The statistical hypothesis is also referred to as the null hypothesis because it is stated in the null form—that is, a statement of no difference between the variables. This statement may not reflect the outcome expected by the researcher, and thus may cause much confusion to the beginning researcher. It is used as a part of the decision making procedures, which are statistically based, and

---

11. *Ibid.,* p. 66.

exists because present statistical procedures generally cannot test the research hypothesis directly. As an example, in the following research hypothesis stated in the declarative form, the researcher predicts the outcome of the study: "Primiparas who receive individualized instruction on breast feeding will have a more successful breast feeding experience in their home setting than primiparas who receive group instruction on breast feeding." The following statistical hypothesis, stated in the null (no difference) form, does not reflect the outcome which is really expected by the researcher: "There will be no significant difference in the breast feeding experience in their home setting between primiparas who receive individualized instruction on breast feeding and primiparas who receive group instruction on breast feeding."

Many researchers prefer to state the hypothesis in the null form because to them it reflects a more objective and scientific statement of the relationship between the variables. Also, the requirements of the statistical procedures they plan to use to test the hypotheses may require the null form in order to determine whether an observed relationship is probably a chance relationship (due to sampling error, for example) or is probably a true relationship. However, the null form of the hypothesis rarely reflects the researcher's true prediction of the study's outcome, and statements in the null form make it difficult to tie the hypothesis back to the background and theory of the research. Other researchers, therefore, prefer to use the research hypothesis, in which case the underlying null hypothesis is usually assumed without being explicitly stated.

Gay [12] suggests a general paradigm or model for stating research hypotheses (predictions of differences between variables) for experimental studies which we find useful:

X's who get Y do better on Z than X's who do not get Y (Or get some other Y)

---

12. L. R. Gay, *Educational Research: Competencies for Analysis and Application* (Columbus, Ohio: Charles E. Merrill 1976), p. 39.

In this model, X's are the subjects

   Y is the treatment (independent variable)
   Z is the observed outcome (dependent variable)

As an example, "Primiparas (X's or subjects) who receive individualized instruction on breast feeding (Y, the treatment) will have a more successful breast feeding experience in their home setting (Z, observed outcome) than primiparas who receive group instruction (get some other Y, treatment)."

When this model is applied to the null hypothesis previously stated, it looks like this: "There will be no significant difference in the breast feeding experience in their home setting (Z, expected outcome) between primiparas (X's, subjects) who receive individualized instruction on breast feeding (Y, the treatment) and primiparas who receive group instruction on breast feeding (some other Y, treatment)."

Another form for a research hypothesis is the "if . . . then form": "*If* primiparas receive individualized instruction on breast feeding, *then* they will have a more successful breast feeding experience in their homes than primiparas who receive group instruction." Either of these formats should help you write a statement that is truly a hypothesis.

In summary, although a hypothesis may be stated in different ways, the hypothesis statement should be in the form of an answer to the question(s) proposed by the study, state an expressed relationship, be stated clearly and concisely, and be based on an accepted theory and/or valid research findings when possible. It must also be testable, that is, the researcher formulates a hypothesis for a research study in order to accept or to reject it. The researcher must be able to collect and analyze data in such a way as to determine the validity of the hypothesis. Remember, a hypothesis is either supported or rejected, it is never proven or not proven.

You should understand that the success of a research study does not depend on the hypothesis being supported by the data. In a well designed and executed research study, a hypothesis which is not supported can add just as much to the knowledge base, and to the theory from which it was derived, as a well designed and executed study where the hypothesis was supported.

Definition of Terms

Just as the conceptual or theoretical framework and the hypothesis stem from the literature review, so do the definitions of the terms used in the study. The words in the statement of the study's purpose should be defined either directly or operationally. A direct definition uses the definition found in a dictionary.

Operational Definitions

An operational definition provides a full description of the method by which the concept will be studied. This is stated in behavioral, observable, demonstrable terms by citing the *operations* (the manipulation and observations) necessary to produce the phenomenon. For example, in the previously described statement of the purpose of the study, "the purpose of this study is to describe the effect of individualized versus group instruction on successful breast feeding of primiparas in a home setting," the variables to be defined include individualized teaching, group teaching, successful breast feeding in a home setting and primipara. Individual teaching might be defined as a one-to-one instructional relationship between the professional nurse and the primipara. Group teaching might be defined as instruction of several primiparas by the nurse. Successful breast feeding in a home setting might be defined as the degree to which difficulties with home breast feeding were identified as problematic on a questionnaire administered to the mother four months after delivery. These are all operational definitions. *Primipara* can be defined directly by the definition found in a dictionary.

Writing the Problem Statement Section
of a Research Proposal

In this chapter, we discussed the initial step in the research process: the selection and statement of the research problem. The introductory phase of a research proposal entails a discussion of the following elements of the research:

1. Background and rationale for selecting the study problem, including significance of the problem and relevance of the problem to nursing
2. Review of related literature
3. Placing the problem within a conceptual or theoretical framework
4. Statement of the purpose of the study followed by definitions for all the terms used in the statement of the purpose.

In this initial section of the research proposal, the study's general subject area is discussed and then narrowed down to the study's focus. It concludes with the research question which should be stated in declarative form. Enough background material should be presented to acquaint the reader with the problem's importance. The rationale for selecting the problem for study should be discussed as well as the study's significance and its contribution to nursing's scientific knowledge base. If possible, the problem should be placed in a theoretical or conceptual framework and a review of the relevant literature should be presented. The study's purpose should be stated in a clearly defined statement as a declarative sentence, a question, or a hypothesis (hypotheses) to be tested. All terms used should be defined either directly or operationally. The Guidelines for Writing a Research Proposal (Appendix G) should help you to write the problem statement section of your proposal.

The following Application Activities are designed to help you evaluate your understanding of the selection and statement of a research problem.

Application Activities

I Problem Selection
   1. Make a list of at least three general problem areas in nursing that interest you enough to conduct a research study on them.
   2. Narrow each of the above general problem areas to a specific research problem, stated in the form of a question.
   3. Select two of the above research problems and evaluate them in terms of the problem selection criteria presented in this chapter.

II Review of Related Literature
Complete the following exercise designed to familiarize you with a variety of library sources on the research topic you finally decide to investigate.[13]
   1. List as many key words as you can that might relate to your nursing research topic. For example, for the topic "breast feeding" the following key words could be related:
   Infants: feeding
   Nutrition: infant nutrition
   Newborn
   Neonatal
   Nursing
   Lactation
   Milk
   Pregnancy
   Bottle feeding
   "Mothering"
   "Feminism"
   2. List three complete references from *Cumulative Index to Nursing Literature* concerning your topic.

---

13. Adapted from: Patricia Dempsey, "Improving Basic Library Skills," *Nursing Research* 26 (September/October 1977):390. Copyright © 1977, American Journal of Nursing Company. Reproduced, with permission, from *Nursing Research,* September/October, Vol. 26, No. 5.

3. Go to *Index Medicus* and list two complete references related to your topic.
4. Using *Excerpta Medica,* list two complete references related to your topic.
5. List one complete reference from *Dissertation Abstracts* related to your topic.
6. Using *Psychological Abstracts* to locate psychological studies related to your topic, list at least two complete references from this source.
7. List at least three books which relate to your topic (include author, title, publication date, and library call number).
8. Look in *Child Development Abstracts* to determine pediatric applications of your topic.
9. Are there any geriatric implications for your topic?
10. List at least two references from *Nursing Research* related to your topic.
11. Are there references related to your topic in:
    a. *Hospital Literature Index?*
    b. *International Nursing Index?*
    c. *Readers' Guide to Periodical Literature?*
12. List at least three references from Government Documents related to your topic.
13. There are many other abstracts and indices available which might provide additional reference citations related to your topic.
    a. List at least four abstracts and indices related to your topic in addition to those you have already used.
    b. Cite one reference related to your topic from each of the abstracts or indices you have listed above.
14. Investigate your media center regarding audio-visual holdings concerning the broad area of nursing:
    a. List the names of three films
    b. List the names of three videotapes
    c. List the names of three film loops
    d. List the names of three audio tapes
    e. List the names of three film strips

15. Investigate a computerized literature search available to you through your library or other sources.

III The Purpose of the Study Stated as a Hypothesis

1. Formulate a testable hypothesis on your research problem in both the research and the statistical formats.
2. Can you identify the independent and dependent variables in your hypothesis?

IV Writing the Problem Statement Section of Your Research Proposal

1. Reread the proposals written by beginning researchers (Appendices B, C, D), with special attention to the problem statement sections which include all of the material to the plan for data collection (or methodology) section of their proposals.
2. Utilizing the information and procedures presented in the chapter and the Guidelines in Appendix G, write a tentative first draft of the problem statement section of your own proposal which includes:
   a. Statement of the problem including background and significance to nursing
   b. Review of related literature
   c. Placement of the problem within a conceptual or theoretical framework, if possible
   d. Statement of the purpose of the study
   e. Definition of terms

Although you will no doubt revise this material later, much of it will be the initial section of your final research proposal.

Bibliography and Suggested Readings

Abdellah, Faye and Levine, Eugene. *Better Patient Care Through Nursing Research,* 2nd ed. New York: The Macmillan Co., 1979.

American Nurses' Association. *Human Rights Guidelines for Nurses in Clinical and Other Research.* Code No. D-465M. Kansas City: The Association, 1975.

———. "The Nurse in Research: ANA Guidelines on Ethical Values," *American Journal of Nursing,* 68 (July 1968): 1504–1507.

———. *Priorities for Research in Nursing.* Code No. D-513M. Kansas City: The Association, May, 1976.

Arminger, Sister Bernadette. "Ethics of Nursing Research: Profile, Principles, Perspective," *Nursing Research,* 26 (September–October 1977):330–336.

Benoliel, Jeanne Q., "The Interaction between Theory and Research," *Nursing Outlook,* 25 (February 1977):108–113.

Brink, Pamela J. and Wood, Marilynn. *Basic Steps in Planning Nursing Research.* North Scituate: Duxbury Press, 1978.

Dempsey, Patricia, "Improving Basic Library Skills," *Nursing Research,* 26 (September–October 1977):390.

de Tornyay, Rheba, "Nursing Research—The Road Ahead," *Nursing Research,* 26 (November–December 1977): 404–407.

Fox, David J. *Fundamentals of Research in Nursing.* 3rd ed. New York: Appleton-Century-Crofts, 1976.

Gay, L. R. *Educational Research: Competencies for Analysis and Application.* Columbus: Charles E. Merrill Publishing Co., 1976.

Holaday, B. J., "Achievement Behavior in Chronically Ill Children," *Nursing Research* 23 (January–February 1974):25–30.

Jacox, A., "Theory Construction in Nursing," *Nursing Research* 23 (January–February 1974):4–13.

Johnson, D. E., "Development of Theory: A Requisite for Nursing as a Primary Health Profession," *Nursing Research* 23 (September–October 1974):372–377.

National League for Nursing. *Theory Development: What, Why, How?* New York: NLN Publication No. 15-1708, 1978.

Stillman, M. J., "Women's Health Beliefs about Breast Cancer and Breast Self-Examination," *Nursing Research* 26 (March–April 1977):121–127.

Van Dalen, D. B. *Understanding Education Research*. New York: McGraw-Hill Book Co., 1973.

Verhonick, Phyllis. *Nursing Research I*. Boston: Little, Brown and Co., 1975.

Verhonick, Phyllis and Seaman, Catherine. *Research Methods for Undergraduate Students in Nursing*. New York: Appleton-Century-Crofts, 1978.

4

Data Collection

I N previous chapters we have presented material on the application of the research process to nursing problems. In the problem selection and statement step of the research process, a researchable problem is selected for study. The material in this chapter is designed to acquaint you with the next step in the research process: development of the overall plan to collect the information directly related to the study problem.

The Nature of Data

The data (information) needed to answer the study question or problem can be classified in two major areas: qualitative data and quantitative data. Research studies can be designed to collect both types of data.

Qualitative Data

Qualitative data are characterized by words (pale; cyanotic; jaundiced). Descriptions in narrative forms and verbatim statements of subjects are examples of qualitative data. They should be used very selectively because this type of data tends to be subjective and lacks the precision that characterizes quantitative data. For example, "several patients were admitted to the CCU early yesterday afternoon" is not as precise as "two patients were admitted to the CCU at 1 P.M. yesterday (April 12, 1979)."

Quantitative Data

Quantitative data are characterized by numbers (temperature $= 98.6°F$; $B/P = 120/90$). The ability to quantify data enhances the precision of the study. It is possible to convert qualitative data to quantitative data by measuring the variables. This can be done with an instrument that allows the investigator to assign numerical values in varying degrees to the existing variable. One of the ways this is frequently done is to quantify the degrees of agreement with a statement on an interview schedule or questionnaire: strongly agree $= 4$; agree $= 3$; disagree $= 2$; strongly disagree $= 1$. This makes it possible to manipulate the numbers when analyzing the responses. Numbers have the advantage of being easier to work with and manipulate than words. Using numbers facilitates the collection of data; their analysis is also facilitated in that numbers are amenable to statistical analysis techniques. Finally, the investigator can objectively compare the data generated by the study with that generated by previous investigators (even in a foreign language), thus placing the current study within the framework of previous knowledge.

Continuous and Discrete Data

You will hear the terms continuous data and discrete data used to refer to quantitative variables. Continuous data can be located at some point along a continuum or scale, and are characterized by fractional values of a whole unit. For example, 98.6°F. body temperature is a point on the Fahrenheit scale used to measure body temperature. Discrete data, on the other hand, exists only in distinct units expressed as whole numbers that are precise and definite: 6 patients, 5 hospitals, 6 beds rather than $6\frac{1}{2}$ patients, $5\frac{1}{4}$ hospitals or $6\frac{2}{3}$ beds.

The decision as to which form to use to collect data depends upon the nature of the study's research approach, and the need for precision, as well as the availability of appropriate data collection instruments. One of the problems with quantification is the lack of instruments for collecting quantitative data. Nursing research is often concerned with such areas of study as wellness, illness, reactions to various situations, and so forth, which are not easily amenable to quantified measurements.

In general, planning to collect data in quantitative form provides a more functional approach and helps you manipulate the data for analysis.

The Research Approach

In Chapter 1, we stated that the research approaches most commonly used can be classified as: (1) descriptive (also termed survey); (2) experimental (also termed explanatory); and (3) historical (also termed documentary).

Differences between Research Approaches

These approaches are differentiated mainly by their time orientation and the extent to which the investigator has control over manipulating the independent variable. The historical approach is *past oriented* as it examines what was and the investigator has no control over manipulating the independent variable. The descriptive approach is *present oriented* as it describes what is and the investigator has no control over manipulating the independent variable. The experimental approach is *future oriented* in predicting what will be; here the investigator has control over manipulating the independent variable in the experimental setting.

The table on page 67 summarizes these characteristic differences between the approaches.

Selecting the Research Approach

You will also see the research approaches referred to as *research methods* or *research designs*. All of these terms refer to the *overall plan* for eliciting information on the study problem. You will remember that the research process has been described as a chain of reasoning beginning with the

Research Approach	Time Orientation	Control of Independent Variable by Investigator
Historical	Past (examining "what was")	No
Descriptive	Present (describing "what is")	No
Experimental	Future (predicting "what will be")	Yes

statement of the problem and systematically proceeding through to communication of the study results. From this it is evident that the statement of the problem section of the research plan will guide the choice of the study's research approach. An important consideration is the extent to which the research problem fits the framework of existing knowledge and theory. Use of the experimental approach requires more extensive knowledge, that the problem be formulated within a conceptual or theoretical framework, and the ability to predict the action of the variables.[1]

The form in which the purpose of the study is stated also guides the choice of the research approach. In general, the declarative statement and the question indicate a descriptive or historical approach, while the hypothesis indicates an experimental approach because the investigator has control over manipulating the independent variable.[2] While it is possible to have a hypothesis in the historical and descriptive approaches, it is not tested by direct manipulation of the variables as in the experimental setting, but by statistical manipulation of already existing data.

Thus, in the step-by-step chain of reasoning that characterizes the research process, the components of the statement

1. Pamela Brink and Marilynn Wood, *Basic Steps in Planning Nursing Research* (North Scituate: Duxbury Press, 1978), chart following Preface, n. p.
2. *Ibid.*

of the problem and the form of the statement of the purpose guide the selection of the research approach. The proposal reprinted in Appendix D can be used to illustrate these principles. The investigator planned to study the effect of kinetic nursing (the independent variable) on the respiratory status of immobilized patients by analyzing (the dependent variable) arterial blood gas values. Her choice of the experimental research approach was guided by the main components of the problem statement, which included a fairly extensive discussion of knowledge related to the topic and an elaboration of the concept of kinetic nursing. The investigator predicts the action of the variables (predicts what will be) in the purpose of the study stated here as a null hypothesis: "The purpose of this study will be to test the following hypothesis: In the neurosurgical intensive care unit at a large county hospital there will be no significant change in immobilized patients' arterial blood gas values when the Roto-Rest Bed is temporarily stopped." Notice that the investigator has control over manipulating the independent variable in the experimental setting in that the effect of kinetic nursing is defined as any immobilized patient being treated on the Roto-Rest Bed.

Data Gathering Techniques

We have seen that the research approach refers to the overall method for obtaining the study's data. Choice of the techniques for gathering the data depends on the nature and sources of the data to be collected. Many research studies utilize more than one technique for gathering data. For example, in a study designed to describe the learning achieved by student nurses on caring for terminally ill patients, learning could be measured in the cognitive, affective, and psychomotor domains. A paper and pencil test could be used to gather data measuring cognitive learning (knowledge); an interview schedule could be used to ascertain attitudes on the affective domain; and an observational check list could be used to gather data on the student's technical proficiency in performing psychomotor skills (procedures).

Characteristics of Research Instruments

When we refer to research instruments or research tools, we are talking about the devices or equipment used to gather the research data. Research instruments must possess certain basic attributes; these assure us that they will provide dependable measurement of the variables under investigation. The most important attributes are (1) validity; (2) reliability; (3) usability.

Validity

Validity refers to the ability of a data gathering instrument to measure what it is supposed to measure, that is, to obtain data relevant to what is being measured. Validity is the most important characteristic of a measuring instrument. A clinical thermometer is a valid instrument for measuring an individual's body temperature, but a sphygmomanometer is not valid for this purpose. A yardstick is a valid instrument for measuring yards of cloth, whereas a baby scale is obviously not a valid instrument for this measurement. In estimating the validity of a measuring instrument, the questions "Valid for what?" and "Valid for whom?" must be answered. In the case of measuring body temperature, the clinical thermometer is valid for measuring body temperature (what?) on human beings, blood vertebrates (whom?).

There are two main approaches for estimating the validity of a measuring instrument: *logical validity* and *statistical validity*. Logical validity is determined primarily through logic or judgment. Statistical validity is determined through appropriate statistical measures.

LOGICAL VALIDITY Logical validity consists of two main types: (1) *face validity,* and (2) *content validity. Face validity* for a measuring instrument is determined by inspecting the items to see if the instrument contains important items which measure the variables in the content area. Face validity is subjective and is the least time consuming and the least rigorous method of determining validity.

Content validity of a measuring instrument deals with the extent to which the instrument represents the factors under study. Content validity is determined by expert judgment. That is, a number of experts in the field of the specific study topic are requested to assess the content validity of the instrument. Members of this expert panel then examine each item and make judgments regarding how well the items reflect the congruity between what is actually included and what should be included. There are no statistical procedures involved in determining the content validity of a measuring instrument.

STATISTICAL VALIDITY In contrast to logical validity where no statistical procedures are involved, *statistical validity* utilizes statistical procedures to estimate validity. There are three types of statistical validity: (1) *Construct*, (2) *Concurrent*, and (3) *Predictive*.

Construct validity can be defined as the degree to which a measuring instrument measures a specific hypothetical construct, such as intelligence. *Concurrent validity* is the degree to which scores on a measuring instrument are related to the scores on an already existing measuring instrument of known validity which is administered at the same time. *Predictive validity* is the degree to which a measuring instrument is able to predict how well the individual will perform in some future situation.[3] (Procedures for estimating statistical validity can be found in statistics books and more advanced research methodology books.)

In summary, logical validity is determined primarily

---

3. L. R. Gay, *Educational Research: Competencies for Analysis and Application* (Columbus: Charles E. Merrill Publishing Co., 1976) 88–91.

through judgment, whereas statistical validity utilizes appropriate statistical measures. Although not as scientific or rigorous as statistical validity, logical validity is more often used in behavioral science research because of the problems associated with estimating validity by statistical methods.

Reliability

The reliability of a measuring instrument refers to its ability to obtain consistent results when reused. An instrument is reliable when it consistently does whatever it is supposed to do the same way every time it is used. For example, when a paper and pencil test of intelligence is administered to a person, it should produce approximately the same result if it is readministered as a retest at a later date. The more reliable a measuring instrument is, the more confidence we can have that the scores obtained would not fluctuate too greatly from administration time to administration time.

Reliability is usually expressed as a number, called a coefficient. A high coefficient indicates high reliability. A measuring instrument that has perfect reliability has a coefficient of 1.00. However, rarely is a measuring instrument perfectly reliable. Reliability is more often reported as less than 1.00, that is, .80, .70, or .50. A correlation coefficient of .80 is usually considered to be an acceptable level of reliability for the measuring instruments using the types of reliability we will be discussing.[4] Less than perfect reliability of an instrument is due to errors in measurement, such as the conditions under which the test was administered (improper directions), problems with the instrument itself (poorly constructed items), or by characteristics of the persons responding to the instrument (illness or fatigue).

There are several main types of reliability which are determined through correlation: (1) *test–retest reliability,* (2) *alternate forms reliability,* and (3) *split–half reliability.*

---

4. Brink, p. 126.

TEST–RETEST RELIABILITY This type indicates variation in scores from one administration of the instrument to the next resulting from measurement errors. The procedure for determining test–retest reliability is to administer the instrument to individuals similar to the ones you plan to study, let a period of time elapse (say a week) to allow for some loss of memory for the items, then give the instrument to the same individuals again. The scores on the two instruments are then correlated statistically to yield a coefficient referred to as the coefficient of stability. If the results are the same or similar, the coefficient will be high—say .90—and the instrument is said to have high test–retest reliability. One of the major problems with this method of estimating reliability is realistically deciding how long the time interval between the test and the retest should be. If the time interval is too short, the individuals tend to remember their responses to the items on the first administration. This results in an artificially high coefficient of reliability. If the time interval is too long, some individuals may not be available for the retest. Also, individuals may do better on a retest because of their own learning and maturation during the interval between the test and the retest.

ALTERNATE FORMS RELIABILITY This is also called equivalent forms reliability. In this type at least two different forms of the instrument are constructed. Although the actual items on the instruments are not the same, each form has the same total number of test items, is designed to measure the same variable or variables, and has the same level of difficulty. Both use the same procedures for administration, scoring, and interpreting the results. At least two different forms of the instrument must be available. The procedure for determining alternate forms reliability is to administer one form of the test to the individuals; then, at the same session or very shortly after, administer a second form to the same individuals. The two sets of scores are then statistically correlated and the instrument has good alternate forms reliability if the correlation coefficient is high. There are two

major problems with this method. One is the difficulty involved in constructing two forms which are equivalent; this
can result in measurement errors. The second is the difficulty
in administering two different instruments to the same individuals within a relatively short time period.

SPLIT–HALF RELIABILITY   This form is also called odd–even
reliability and the coefficient of internal consistency. This
estimate of reliability requires only one administration of
an instrument in order to estimate its reliability. The entire
instrument is administered to the individuals, then the responses for each individual are divided into two comparable
halves: all the responses to even items in one half, and all
the responses to odd items in the other half. The response
score for each individual is then computed separately for
the two halves, resulting in a response score for the even
items and a response score for the odd items. The two sets
of scores are then correlated statistically to yield a correlation coefficient. If this is high, the instrument is said to
have good split–half reliability. This method is more effective for longer instruments. For an instrument consisting of
a limited number of items, a correlation formula, such as the
Spearman-Brown prophecy formula must be applied. The
split–half method of estimating reliability has the advantage
of requiring only one administration and one form of the
instrument; it also eliminates the problems associated with
more than one administration of the instrument to the same
individuals.

Usability

The usability of a measuring instrument refers to the practical aspects of using it. These include ease of administration,
scoring, and interpretation as well as financial, time and
energy considerations. It is important to an instrument's
reliability and validity that these practical aspects be considered.

In summary, the basic attributes that characterize dependable research instruments, or tools, are: (1) validity, (2) reliability, and (3) usability. Since the outcome of a research study depends on the instrument(s) used to collect the data, research instruments that meet these criteria increase the potential for high quality research.

Considerations in Selecting a Measuring Instrument

Since it takes a great deal of time and skill to develop your own instrument, it is better to select an appropriate instrument that has already been developed. If you are fortunate enough to locate an instrument that appears to measure what you want, keep looking and try to compare more than one tool on relevant factors. The sources of instrument compilations listed in Chapter 3 may help you locate instruments appropriate for your study.

If you have to use a self-developed measuring instrument, you can take parts of one or more instruments to develop it. Do not plan to use a self-developed instrument unless you pretest the instrument on a group similar to the one to be used in your study. A pretest is the process of testing out the effectiveness of the instrument in gathering the appropriate data. The instrument is administered to subjects who meet the criteria for study subjects, and the investigator evaluates its strengths and weaknesses and revises it as necessary.

Selecting the Study Subjects

An essential part of the data collection plan is the selection of the study subjects that will provide the necessary data in relation to the purpose of the study.

The Target Population

The investigator must delineate a *target population* consisting of individual people or things that meet the designated set of criteria of interest to the researcher. In nursing research, the target population usually consists of human beings. However, it can also consist of human characteristics (personality, job activities), inanimate objects, such as hospitals, as well as abstract concepts, such as professional ethics, community attitudes, and so on.[5]

The Sample

Since it is often not feasible to study the whole population directly for reasons such as size, cost, time, or lack of accessibility, a study is usually done on a smaller part of a target population, called a *sample*. The term sampling refers to the process of selecting a number of individuals from the delineated target population in such a way that the individuals in the sample represent (as nearly as possible) the characteristics of the whole target population. The sample can be thought of as a miniature of the larger target population. A single unit or member of the target population is referred to as a population element or a sampling unit.

For example, a study proposes to investigate the effect of educational preparation on the political perceptions of all licensed nurses in the state of Florida. The target population would be all of the licensed nurses in Florida. Since it would probably not be feasible to study such a large number of individuals, a sample of these nurses would be selected for inclusion in the study. This would be done in such a way that they would be representative of all the licensed nurses in Florida. Such a selection could be accomplished by first obtaining a computer listing of all the licensed nurses in the state from the Florida Board of Nursing. The investigator would then select a fraction of the licensed nurses on the list in such a way that those selected for inclusion in the study would be representative of all licensed nurses in Florida. Each licensed nurse in the sample would then be a population element and a sampling unit.

---

5. Faye Abdellah and Eugene Levine, *Better Patient Care through Nursing Research.* 2nd ed. (New York: Macmillan, 1979), p. 152.

Purpose of Sampling

A basic purpose of sampling is to be able to use the sample's findings to say something about the target population, that is, to be able to generalize or extrapolate beyond the actual sampling units without having to study each element of the target population. The extent of this ability to generalize beyond the actual sampling units to the target population depends on the sampling approach used.

Sampling Approaches

Sampling theory distinguishes between two main approaches to sampling: *probability sampling* and *nonprobability sampling*.

PROBABILITY SAMPLING Here the investigator is able to specify, for each element of the population, the probability that it will be included in the sample. Usually, each element has the *same* probability of being included in the sample but the basic requirement is that there exists a *known* probability that it will be included. The sampling units are selected by chance and neither the investigator nor the population elements has any conscious influence on what is included in the sample.

NONPROBABILITY SAMPLING Here the investigator has no ability to estimate the probability that each element of the population will be included in the sample, or even that it has some chance of being included.

The importance of the ability to estimate probability lies in the interpretation of the study findings. Probability sampling has the advantage of permitting the investigator to generalize from the sample's findings to the target population with a given degree of certainty. That is, these sample findings do not differ by more than a specific amount from the findings using the total population. Nonprobability samples do not permit generalization of the study findings from the sample to the population.

Choice of the sampling approach depends on the research problem and the purpose of the study. Not all studies
are conducted with the purpose of being able to generalize
to the population. The important point is that the sampling
approach must be consistent with the purpose of the study.

Probability Sampling Methods

Major methods of probability sampling include: (1) *simple
random sampling;* (2) *stratified random sampling;* and (3)
cluster sampling. The following discussion of each is intended to provide you with an overview of these sampling
methods. You will need to refer to sources on more advanced
research methodology for detailed procedures.

SIMPLE RANDOM SAMPLING   In this method, the required
number of sampling units is selected at random from the
population in such a manner that each population element
has an equal chance (probability) of being selected for the
sample. Each choice of a sampling unit must be independent
of all other choices. One of the most acceptable methods for
selecting a simple random sample is to use a table of random
numbers which can be found in statistics books. The numbers in a table of random numbers have been generated in
such a way that there is no sequencing pattern. The same
probability exists that any digit will follow any other digit
and each selection was an independent choice. Figure 4–1
shows an excerpt from a table of random numbers.

To obtain a simple random sample, first list each of
the population elements, then assign consecutive numbers
to each of these elements. Then, referring to a table of random numbers, start at any point in the table and proceed
in any direction to identify enough tabled numbers to associate with the population elements, thus achieving the desired sample size.

Rather than using a table of random numbers, it is also
possible to select a simple random sample by drawing numbers from a box. The names are placed in a container on

Figure 4–1 Excerpt From a Table of Random Numbers

57	87	59	93	27
86	05	14	21	98
04	67	95	16	47
11	37	31	34	22
27	16	20	26	62
87	22	50	14	55
00	34	33	21	24
47	14	30	62	50
67	96	51	49	40
43	80	44	48	62
90	52	60	28	86
51	92	99	77	98
26	64	77	32	29
20	34	47	55	69
81	45	58	72	83
83	80	73	19	77
80	33	14	76	93
40	93	76	82	83
55	52	48	67	21
15	87	46	87	92
06	03	21	27	71
07	68	15	05	64
84	59	73	39	87
75	33	18	30	12

folded pieces of paper and mixed well. The first name chosen is assigned to the sample, but because the probability associated with subsequent choices is not constant, the slip should be replaced in the container each time a name is selected to more fully approach random selection. This procedure is called sampling with replacement, and is not as rigorous as using a table of random numbers in that each choice of a sampling unit is not independent of all other choices—once it is chosen, it will not be included in the sample again.

One of the problems in using simple random sampling is the difficulty in obtaining or compiling a list of each of the population elements, either because they are not known or the size of the listing proves to be prohibitive for a large population.

STRATIFIED RANDOM SAMPLE   This method is a variation of the simple random sample. The population is divided into two or more strata, or different categories of a characteristic. A simple random sample is then taken from each group. This procedure is used when the composition of the population is known with respect to some characteristic or characteristics. The variables (characteristics) chosen to stratify the population must be important to the study. For example, a population of 500 human elements may be stratified on the basis of sex. Then, one half of the sampling units may be chosen from the female category and the other half from the male category by simple random sampling. This assures that the sample will consist of equal allocation from each population stratum. A population may be divided into other strata or categories, such as age, educational background, occupation, and so on.

The basic purpose of selecting random samples—either simple or stratified—is to permit the investigator to utilize appropriate inferential statistical procedures. These depend on random selection and allow the investigator to make generalizations from the sample results to the study population.

CLUSTER SAMPLING   A method also known as multistage sampling, cluster sampling is used in large-scale studies in which the population is geographically spread out. The cluster is the primary sampling unit and consists of groups, rather than individuals, all of whom have the same characteristic. For example, a cluster could consist of nursing homes, or hospitals, or schools of nursing as the primary sampling units. In subsequent sampling stages, a random sample of the various nursing units in each hospital could be taken, then the third stage could sample the patients on whom the actual measurements are needed for the study.[6] Cluster sampling has the advantage of convenience, and involves less time and

---

6. *Ibid.*, p. 329.

money in large-scale studies while retaining the advantages of probability sampling.

The term systematic sampling is used to refer to the selection of sampling units by taking every Kth name on a population list, such as every 4th name listed on a hospital census sheet. Systematic sampling is considered a method of probability sampling *only if* the population list is randomly ordered and each population element has a known probability of being included in the sample.

Nonprobability Sampling Methods

In nonprobability sampling, the investigator has no ability to estimate the probability that each element of the population will be included in the sample. Major methods of nonprobability sampling include: (1) convenience samples, (2) purposive samples, and (3) quota samples.

CONVENIENCE SAMPLING   This method is also called accidental sampling. The sampling units are selected simply because they are available—they are in the right place at the right time for the investigator's purposes. For example, in the investigation of the effects of kinetic nursing on immobilized patients' blood gas values (Appendices D, E) the investigator selected a convenience sample including the first 10 patients admitted to the neurosurgical intensive care unit and placed on the Roto-Rest Bed as of January 1, 1979.

PURPOSIVE SAMPLING   This method is also called judgment sampling. The investigator establishes certain criteria and the sampling units are selected according to these criteria. For example, in the research proposal in Appendix C, the investigator planned to use a purposive sample consisting of specific criteria in regard to physician, hospital, maternity unit, age and family placement of infant, medical complications, and so on.

QUOTA SAMPLING   This method is much like convenience sampling, but certain controls are established so that the sample does not become overloaded with subjects having certain characteristics. The investigator specifies a percentage for each characteristic to be in each group so that it is proportionate to the characteristics of the population. For example, a Gallup Poll may use quota sampling to assure that males and females from certain age, ethnic, and occupational groups are represented in the sample in proportion to these characteristics in the population.

Although it is often difficult to obtain probability samples in clinical research, both probability and nonprobability sampling have a respected place in research—neither is better than the other. The important factor in determining which sampling approach to use is consistency with the research problem and the study's purpose.

Sample Size

In determining how many subjects to include in a study (the total N for the study), it may be feasible to collect data regarding each element of the population. More often, however, the investigator will need to sample from the target population, and is faced with the decision of how large a sample will produce sufficient data to fulfill the study's purpose. There are no simple rules for determining sample size. It is primarily determined by the degree of precision required, the type of sampling procedure used, the homogeneity of the population, as well as cost and convenience factors. A general rule is to use as large a sample as possible within feasible constraints. The larger the number in the sample, the more likely it will be representative of the population from which it was selected. Representativeness of the sample is an important concern:

> The question of how large a sample should be is basically unanswerable, other than to say that it should be large enough to achieve representativeness.[7]

---

7. David J. Fox, *Fundamentals of Research in Nursing.* 3rd ed. (New York: Appleton-Century-Crofts, 1976), p. 175.

In general, the larger the sample, the more generalizable the study results. If the population is homogeneous, a smaller sample size may be adequate.

We have found the following general guidelines helpful in determining sample size:

1. A sample of 10% of the population is considered minimum for descriptive studies, and a minimum of 15 subjects per group for experimental studies.[8]
2. It is advisable to include at least 5, preferably more, sampling units for each category of each variable in order to have enough data to analyze.

Even with these general guidelines, the investigator should bear the following in mind:

A large sample cannot correct for a faulty sampling design. The researcher should make decisions about sample size and design with the following in mind: the ultimate criterion for assessing a sample is its representativeness, not the quantity of data it produces.[9]

In summary, the method of selecting subjects for the study must be consistent with the problem and purpose of the study and involves identification of the target population. If sampling is indicated, the sample should be of sufficient size to be representative of the population and provide sufficient data for analysis. The sampling approach (probability or nonprobability) must also be consistent with the research design.

Stating the Assumptions of the Study

An assumption is a statement whose correctness or validity is taken for granted. Assumptions may be so self-

8. L. R. Gay, p. 77.
9. Denise Polit and Bernadette Hungler, *Nursing Research: Principles and Methods* (Philadelphia: J. B. Lippincott Co., 1978) p. 467.

evident as to require no further testing, they may be based on theories applicable to the study topic, or they may be based on previous research findings.[10] In most studies, assumptions are implied by the investigator and need not be stated explicitly. If they are significant enough to affect the study's course or outcome, the investigator should state these assumptions explicitly so that others may evaluate their effect on the study.

Stating the Limitations of the Study

Limitations of the study are restrictions that may affect the investigator's ability to generalize the study results and over which the investigator has no control. Although all studies are limited in some way, limitations are usually related to the use of small, unrepresentative samples and inadequate methodology. Important limitations should be stated, both in the research proposal and the research report, to allow the reader to judge their effect on the study.

Writing the Data Collection Section of a Research Proposal

In this chapter, we discussed principles and methods on the development of the overall plan to collect the data on the study problem. The data collection section of a research proposal consists of a discussion of the following topics on the plan for collecting the data:

1. The research approach
2. Plans for selecting the study subjects (sampling)
3. Techniques for data collection
4. Procedures for data collection

---

10. Abdellah, p. 145.

5. Assumptions for the study
6. Limitations of the study

In writing this section of the research proposal, the re-search approach is described as either historical, descriptive (survey) or experimental. Plans for selection of the study subjects are specified in terms of a description of the target population, kinds and numbers of study subjects, and the sampling approach and method (if applicable). Techniques for collecting the data are described in relation to the study's purpose, and measuring instruments are described and dis-cussed in terms of their reliability, validity, and usability. An experimental study should also include a description of the experimental design. Steps in the procedure for data collection should be listed in chronological order with atten-tion to the protection of human rights. Any explicit assump-tions that would significantly affect the study should be stated. Finally, limitations of the study should be listed. The guidelines for writing a research proposal (Appendix G) should help you write this section of your proposal.

The following application activities are designed to help you evaluate your understanding of principles and proce-dures on data collection.

Application Activities

I Selecting the Research Approach
  1. Reread the research study reprinted in Appendix A with special attention to the research approach and method of data collection.
     a. Explain how the study's purpose (to test the research hypothesis) directed the selection of the research ap-proach.
     b. Describe how the study has a future time orientation (predicting "what will be").
     c. Identify the independent variable (the treatment) and the dependent variable (the result or the effect).
     d. Discuss the ways in which the investigators had control of the independent variable in the research setting.

II Selecting the Study Subjects
1. Refer again to the research study reprinted in Appendix A.
   a. Is the target population described? How?
   b. Explain why the study subjects are referred to as a population, rather than a sample.
   c. Discuss the relationship of each of the criteria for selection of the study subjects to the study's purpose.
   d. Describe how the study subjects were selected and then assigned to experimental and control groups.
   e. How many subjects were included in the study (N = ___)?
2. The desired sample size for a study is 20 subjects to be selected from a target population of 40 elements. Select the subjects to be included in the sample by the following procedure:
   a. List the elements (names) of the target population.
   b. Number the names consecutively from 01 to 20.
   c. Arbitrarily select a 2 digit column from the excerpt of a table of random numbers in this chapter (Figure 4-1).
   d. When a number corresponds to a number assigned to a name on the list of the target population, assign that name to the sample.
   e. Skip any number which is not from 01 to 40 and go on to the next number.
   f. Continue to select each two-digit number that corresponds to the list of names until 20 names have been assigned to the sample.

III Criteria for Evaluating Measuring Instruments
Locate at least two measuring instruments which might be helpful in collecting data related to some aspect of your study. For each instrument:
   a. Describe how the reliability was established and reported.
   b. Describe how the validity was established and reported.
   c. Discuss the usability for your study.

IV Writing the Data Collection Section of Your Research Proposal
1. Reread the proposals in Appendices B, C, D; pay special attention to the data collection sections of each proposal.

2. Utilizing the principles and procedures in this chapter, and the guidelines in Appendix G, write a tentative first draft of the plan for data collection section of your own proposal which includes:
   a. Description of the research approach
   b. Plan for selecting the study subjects
   c. Techniques for data collection
   d. Procedures for data collection
   e. Assumptions and limitations of the study

Although you will undoubtedly revise some of this material, you should be able to use much of it in your final research proposal.

Bibliography and Suggested Readings

Abdellah, Faye and Levine, Eugene. *Better Patient Care Through Nursing Research*, 2nd ed. New York: The Macmillan Co., 1979.

Brink, Pamela J. and Wood, Marilynn. *Basic Steps in Planning Nursing Research*. North Scituate: Duxbury Press, 1978.

Ford, Julienne. *Paradigms and Fairy Tales*, 2 vols. London: Routledge and Kegan Paul, 1975.

Fox, David. *Fundamentals of Research in Nursing*, 3rd ed. New York: Appleton-Century-Crofts, 1976.

Gay, L. R. *Educational Research: Competencies for Analysis and Application*. Columbus: Charles E. Merrill Publishing Co., 1976.

Hopkins, Charles D. *Educational Research: A Structure for Inquiry*. Columbus: Charles E. Merrill Publishing Co., 1976.

Mouly, G. J. *The Science of Educational Research*, 2nd ed. New York: Litton Educational Publishing Co., 1970.

Notter, Lucille. *Essentials of Nursing Research*, 2nd ed. New York: Springer Publishing Co., 1978.

Polit, Denise and Hungler, Bernadette. *Nursing Research:*

Principles and Methods. New York: J. B. Lippincott Co., 1978.

Selltiz, Claire; Wrightsman, Lawrence; and Cook, S. *Research Methods in Social Relations,* 3rd ed. New York: Holt, Rinehart and Winston, 1976.

Verhonick, Phyllis and Seaman, Catherine. *Research Methods for Undergraduate Students in Nursing.* New York: Appleton-Century-Crofts, 1978.

Wandelt, Mabel. *Guide for the Beginning Researcher.* New York: Appleton-Century-Crofts, 1970.

5

Data Analysis

T HE purpose of this chapter is to acquaint you with some very basic information about the analysis and interpretation of data in research studies; it should help you understand and evaluate the different methods of treating data statistically. We do not intend or require that beginning researchers be statisticians. Consequently, this chapter is intended to be a simplified overview of statistical techniques and analysis. Researchers who need more help in developing statistical analyses are urged to contact their instructors, a statistician, or other qualified individuals.

The Use of Statistics in Data Analysis

Statistics are ways of measuring things or groups of things. Any time we measure opinions, average numbers of miles per gallon, or the odds in a card game, we are using statistics. Basically, there are two kinds of statistics: descriptive and inferential. Descriptive statistics simply describe the population we are concerned with. Inferential statistics allow us to draw other kinds of conclusions about a population, based on a sample or samples, and to predict future happenings.

Descriptive Statistics

Essentially, descriptive statistics describe. This type of statistical analysis is the simple reporting of facts and collective occurrences based on a number of samples.

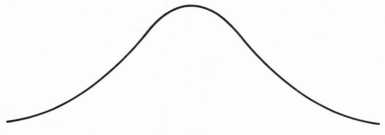

Normal Curve

We are concerned with several types of measures when we use descriptive statistics: (1) centrality or central tendency, (2) dispersion, and (3) location or position within the sample or population.

If you were to measure any large population you would find that the members of the population would distribute themselves across what is known as the normal curve.

The Mean

As you can easily see, most of the population clusters about the high point, or center of the curve. If the curve is perfectly symmetrical, the center of the normal curve is called the mean. Statistically, the mean is shown by the symbol $\overline{X}$. The mean may be thought of as the average.

For example, suppose we have seven scores on a simple test:

$$5, 4, 3, 2, 6, 7, 8$$

When we add these scores and then divide the sum by the total number of tests, we find that 5 is the mean or average in this case.

Of course, means describe essentially mythical characteristics. No one owns 1.3 cars or 2.2 television sets, or has 2.5 children. What the mean does is give us some idea of what a total population may be like, but it is not a measure in which we can put our complete trust. For example, suppose we have seven more scores from a test:

$$6, 7, 8, 5, 4, 10, 23$$

The mean of these seven scores is now 9. Yet only two scores are above 9. This average implies something that is not an accurate reflection of what really happened with the test scores. The curve is distorted.

The Median

When we have such extreme scores that can cause a distortion of the curve, we can utilize another measure that shows how central the mean really is. This is called the median. The median is the number that divides the sample in half. Fifty percent of any sample falls above the median and fifty percent falls below the median. In our first example of seven scores we find that the median is 5. This is the same as the mean. In the second example, however, the median is 7. In this particular instance, 7 is probably more descriptive of what is really happening than the mean of 9.

The Mode

Still another measure of central tendency is the mode. This statistic tells us where scores tend to cluster. For example:

$$4, 5, 6, 6, 6, 7, 8$$

The most frequently occurring score or number is 6. Consequently, the mode is 6. In this example, the mean and the median also happen to be 6.

Remember, it is fairly unusual and inadvisable to use descriptive statistics exclusively with small samples. Such techniques will distort the data analysis.

Percentile Rank

Measures that reflect the relative position of a score in a distribution are also descriptive in nature. One of the most commonly used statistics is the percentile rank. The percentile rank is the point below which a percentage of scores occur. In percentile rank, the median is always the 50th percentile. A person scoring at the 60th percentile is above 60% of the other test takers and below the other 40%.

Other percentage-based statistics commonly found in the literature are the decile (10%) and the quartile (25%).

Means, medians, and modes are used when we want to describe measures of central tendency. They give us an idea of how alike a population is. However, we sometimes want to know how a population is actually distributed over the curve. This means that we must use measures of dispersion. The most frequently used measure of dispersion is the standard deviation.

The Standard Deviation

On all normal curves, certain proportions of the sample cluster around the mean. We can measure how widely distributed the scores are by measuring the standard deviation. When a curve is normal, about 68% of the population will be within one plus or one minus standard deviation of the mean. We discuss the average characteristics of a population when we report the mean, but we usually consider this 68%—34% above the mean and 34% below the mean—to be within the normal or average range.

Ninety-five percent of the population will be within two standard deviations from the mean and ninety-nine and seven-tenths will be within three standard deviations.

The important idea is not the percentages of the population that are contained under any portion of a curve, but

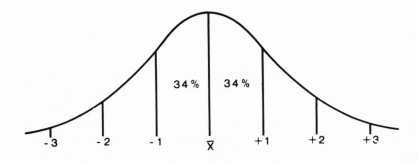

rather the shape of the curve. There is one standard (imaginary) bell shaped curve that we have been using to illustrate the idea of the statistical curve. Curves can take many shapes, however, some with a narrow range and others with a wide range between standard deviations.

If a test is given and the standard deviation is found to be 2 and the mean is 16 this means that 68% of the population will fall between the scores of 14 and 18 on the normal curve. If the standard deviation of the same test is 4, the curve will assume a different shape; if the standard deviation is 8, still another shape will be assumed. Consequently, we can always describe the shape of the curve based on the standard deviation. We can also get some idea of the range of the scores and a better feeling for an average individual.

Inferential Statistics

Descriptive statistics provide us with a quantitative way of viewing the world. That is, we are able to describe certain factual aspects about a population. However, most researchers are concerned with other kinds of judgments as well. This leads us to the use of inferential statistics. Essentially, inferential statistics do not examine a whole population. Rather, as described in Chapter 4, a sample or samples are drawn from the population and the characteristics of the population are deduced or inferred from the responses of the sample.

In addition to this type of inference, the researcher uses inferential statistics to determine whether or not certain experimental treatments or techniques are better, worse, or not significantly different from other types of treatments or techniques. This is called hypothesis testing and is based on probability. When reading research, the beginning researcher continually runs across the proposition $H_0 = p < .05$. Remember that H_0 is called the null hypothesis as discussed in Chapter 3. $p < .05$ is called the level of significance. That is, the researcher states that results will probably *not* be significantly different from the standard or common treatment. Most researchers really want to reject the null hypothesis, but research convention has cast this as the most common type of research treatment. The symbol "p" stands for probability. The probability in this statement is that there will be no conclusion of significant difference between treatments, unless five or fewer treatments out of one hundred have the same result as the original or standard treatment.

When a level of significance is selected, the experimenter is telling the world that chance has little to do with the results of the experiment. Most medically related experiments set extremely high levels of significance; usually one chance in one thousand or less ($p < .001$). In cases of life and death, the chances of error must be diminished as much as possible.

Levels of Measurement

When dealing with inferential statistics, we must be concerned with what are called levels of measurement. Often the researcher works with data represented by responses to questions which can be posed in various ways.

The Nominal Scale

The first level of data measurement is called the nominal level or nominal scale. The responses to this scale deal only with mutually exclusive data. There are no qualifiers. For example, we can classify all people in the world as having blue eyes or brown eyes. If we choose to do this, anyone whose eyes are considered green, grey, or black must be placed in the category blue or brown. Nominal scales deal only with exclusive categories and do not attempt to find gradations between them. The categories are absolute and the mode is the only measure of central tendency.

In nursing research, the nominal scale might be used to determine if pregnancies and abortions occur statistically

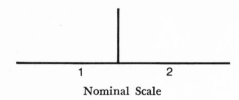

Nominal Scale

more frequently in one of two socially different groups of women. This can be done by simply identifying them as members of one or the other groups and asking them if they have ever had an abortion. The responses of each group could then be tallied and analyzed statistically to determine if there was a significant difference between the two groups.

The Ordinal Scale

The next highest level of measurement is called ordinal measurement. Subjects are asked to rank ideas, items or other things. The subject can respond that item A is more or less than items B or C, but cannot tell exactly how much more or less. For example, a patient may experience more or less discomfort depending on certain postures or other physical phenomena which can be adjusted. The amount cannot really be quantified as saying, "I am twice as uncomfortable," but the feeling of more or less comfort can be experienced. In the previous example, if eye color is graded with a range from black to blue, we could consider this ordinal data and ordinal statistics such as the median would come into play.

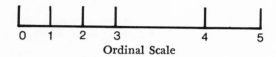

Ordinal Scale

The Interval Scale

The third and most commonly used level of statistical measurement is interval measurement. Actually, much ordinal

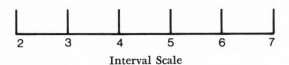

Interval Scale

data is treated as if it were really interval data; there is a great debate in statistical circles as to whether or not this can really be done. Interval measurements are based on absolutely equal distances between measurements. A clinical thermometer is an interval measuring instrument.

The Ratio Scale

The highest level of measurement is the ratio scale. This scale deals with an absolute zero starting point or a base. All subjects start at zero and travel or respond in some manner along this same scale.

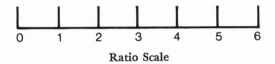

Ratio Scale

Practically speaking, the type of research that is the basis for much of nursing research seldom, if ever, deals with ratio scales.

Commonly Used Statistical Tests

Regardless of scale level used, the researcher must answer the question, "Are the differences I see caused by chance or are other factors, such as my treatment, responsible?" When the researcher sees that two samples have different means, the next task is to test the differences between the means to determine if they are significantly different statistically. Based on the level of data, the researcher selects the statistical test that is the most appropriate to determine if chance is the overriding factor.

t tests

The most commonly used test for determining whether the difference between means is significant is the t test. This allows the researcher to determine whether the difference between the means of two samples is significant and to draw conclusions based on this finding.

Analysis of Variance (ANOVA)

Sometimes the researcher has a series of means to test for a significant difference between them. Then a statistic called analysis of variance or ANOVA is used. With this technique, it is possible to determine if there is a significant difference between several means simultaneously. The literature will report these differences as the F test or F ratio.

Chi Square (χ^2)

The most commonly used test other than the t test is probably the chi square (χ^2). The chi square test is a nonparametric test as opposed to both the t and F tests which are called parametric tests. Nonparametric tests allow the violation of certain assumptions on which parametric tests are based. Essentially, chi squares deal with what can be expected as against what was actually found.

Correlations

Researchers are also concerned about relationships between variables. The relationship between two variables is measured by correlation statistics. This statistic is often expressed by the Pearson r (product-moment correlation coefficient), usually symbolized merely by r. It helps to know that there are a large number of other correlational statistics. Correlational statistics can only range from -1.0 to $+1.0$. It is very important to note that correlations do not imply cause and effect relationships. Correlations that report the presence or absence of something else do not necessarily mean that one caused the other. For example, the correlations between houses with basements and houses with roofs probably approaches +1.0. This does not mean that basements cause roofs. Such a correlation would be a spurious correlation: that is, the assumption of a relationship where none really exists.

Looking at the statistics used in the study reprinted in Appendix A, we find that the data on the treatment of decubitus ulcers with topical application of insulin are analyzed in two ways. First and easiest to read are the tables. Tabular form allows the reader to glance over the data to extract meaning from them. However, merely looking at tables does not provide sufficient information. The data are also discussed in the text of the report. The data are represented in an orderly and meaningful way so that readers can easily understand what was discovered as a result of the research.

A large number of statistical analyses were used in this study. The descriptive techniques of mean, median, mode, standard deviation and range are utilized in order to describe the samples and enhance understanding of the samples' characteristics.

After the samples' characteristics are presented, inferential statistics are used to determine if the differences noted between the groups as a result of the treatment are statistically significant. This report includes the use of analysis of variance (reported as an F ratio), as well as the t test for differences between means and the (Pearson) r. These tests allow the researchers to draw many conclusions about their research; they are presented in the discussion section of the report.

Writing the Data Analysis Section of a Research Proposal

It may seem strange to you that it is important to formulate a plan for data analysis in the planning stage of the research study, and to detail this plan in the research proposal. This assures that the researcher will collect the data in a form that facilitates analysis. The data analysis plan should be appropriate to the problem being investigated and to the methodology of the study. The method of tabulating and organizing the data should be clearly presented as well as a description of appropriate statistical procedures to be applied and the rationale for selecting them.

Skeleton outlines or dummy statistical tables, charts, and graphs will provide a format for analyzing the variables being investigated, and may lead to additional ideas for data analysis. Note that the students who wrote the research proposals included in the appendices established their data collection plan as part of their proposals. Although the best laid plans for data analysis may turn out later to be incomplete or somewhat inappropriate, a carefully formulated plan for data analysis established prior to the actual data collection should result in higher quality research studies. It can also eliminate much distress on the part of the researcher.

The guidelines for writing a research proposal (Appendix G) should help you write this section of your proposal.

A Note on Computers and Calculators

With the advent of computers and hand-held calculators, statistical analysis has become increasingly more sophisticated. This is because many calculations which required hours or days when worked by hand, or on mechanical calculators, can be done in seconds or minutes by the computer or hand calculator with far greater accuracy and fewer mistakes.

Anyone who is serious about research and statistics should acquire a hand calculator. These range from very simple, inexpensive devices to fairly expensive programmable machines. For ease in computation, there are a number of calculators designed to compute the mean, standard deviation and variance. We strongly urge that, at the minimum, any hand calculator you buy has these features.

Most researchers also have access to one or more computers. These machines are technologically very complex and may be intimidating to a beginning researcher. Remember, the computer is simply a tool that can be utilized for data analysis.

There are a number of languages which computers use. Some of these are FORTRAN, BASIC, APL, COBOL and Pascal. Each of these languages is designed to enhance man–machine interaction and to aid in data analysis. It is not necessary, however, for a researcher to know a specific computer language to use the machine. Usually there are teams of consultants who are quite willing and able to help researchers program the machine, and there are many statistical packages which are prewritten and available. One of the most powerful and commonly available sets of programs is the Statistical Package for the Social Sciences (SPSS). This set of programs can deal with almost any kind of data analysis required by most nursing researchers. Another useful set of programs is the Biomedical Data (BMDP).

When initiating a research project that requires analysis by computer, the wise researcher should talk to a computer consultant first in order to cast the data in the easiest form for computer analysis. All computers require that data be put into them in certain ways. Punch cards are used most commonly, but other techniques are available and the researcher should find the easiest method and the most appropriate for the research project.

All researchers would do well to remember the saying, "Garbage In—Garbage Out." The computer can only act on the data given it. If your research is poorly designed, or poorly organized, the finest computer in the world will not provide you with a valid statistical analysis.

There is a great temptation to subject all data to computer analysis just because of the availability of the machine. Frequently, when the number of subjects is small (some say under one hundred), and the statistical computation fairly simple, it is faster and cheaper to do one's calculations by hand. Just setting up a program and removing flaws (debugging) can take a great deal of time. Do not become so enamored of the computer that you waste time trying to use it for all data analysis.

This chapter presented a few basic ideas about statistics and data analysis. Any researcher who wishes to deal in greater depth is strongly urged to take one or more courses in statistics.

Application Activities

Writing the Data Analysis Section of Your Research Proposal
1. Reread the proposals in Appendices B, C, D with special attention to the data analysis sections.
2. Write a tentative first draft of the plan for data analysis section of your own proposal which includes:
   a. A description of the statistical procedures to be used
   b. Dummy charts, graphs, tables as indicated.

Bibliography and Suggested Readings

Cochran, Samuel and Holliman, Joanne. *Cheat Sheet for Stat.* Commerce, Texas, 1974.

Dixon, W. J., ed. *BMDP: Biomedical Computer Programs.* Berkeley: U. of California Press, 1975.

Johnson, Allan G. *Social Statistics without Tears.* New York: McGraw-Hill, 1977.

Malec, Michael A. *Essential Statistics for Social Research.* Philadelphia: J. B. Lippincott, 1977.

Nie, Norman et al. *SPSS: Statistical Package for the Social Sciences,* 2nd ed. New York: McGraw-Hill, 1975.

Siegel, Sidney. *Nonparametric Statistics for the Behavioral Sciences.* New York: McGraw-Hill, 1956.

6

Communicating the Research Results

In the previous chapters we presented material related to Stage I, the *planning stage*, of a research study where the first six steps of the research process were discussed:

1. Statement of the problem
2. Review of related literature
3. Statement of the purpose of the study
4. Definition of the terms
5. Plan for data collection
6. Plan for data analysis

A research proposal is developed by the investigator during the planning stage and provides specific information on these six steps in the research process.

In Stage II of the research study, the *implementation stage*, the investigator puts the research plan into action by collecting the data and anlyzing them in order to determine the study's results.

In Stage III of the research study, the *communication stage*, the investigator interprets the findings, formulates conclusions for the study, and communicates these in the written report of the completed study so that others may share the knowledge. This is the task we will discuss in Chapter 6.

Interpreting the Findings

The data collected in carrying out the study now need to be given meaning by the investigator, who interprets them in terms of the study's purpose. If the study's purpose was to describe certain variables, then meaningful descriptions are indicated. If the study asked a question, the findings should be interpreted to answer this question. If a hypothesis was tested, the study findings should be interpreted as support or rejection of the hypothesis.

Data interpretation is a subjective process; the investigator must be extremely careful not to interpret beyond what the data indicate and must relate conclusions to the study purpose.

Researchers are often hesitant to report negative results of their study. These are results that contradict the theoretical framework, or fail to support the study's hypothesis. In a well designed research study, such results can add as much to existing knowledge as those studies where the results expected by the investigator are produced.

Sometimes a study has important and unexpected findings not related to the original purpose of the study. These are called *serendipitous findings*. The investigator needs to be aware of the possible existence of such findings, and the importance of interpreting and reporting them.

In order to add to existing knowledge, the investigator should also be prepared to relate the study findings to other studies in the same area.

All studies have their own limitations over which the investigator has no control. These limitations and their effect on the interpretation of the data should be discussed.

Finally, since the investigator is the expert on this study, interpretation of the data should result in a discussion of implications for the practice or profession of nursing, and recommendations for further research.

Writing the Research Report

As the final step in the research process, the investigator writes a research report to make the results available and known to others.

Purposes and Characteristics

A research report has several purposes. It may communicate the research results to other investigators, in which case the report should communicate the purpose, procedures, and findings of a study in sufficient detail so that another investigator could replicate the study. In addition, consumers of nursing research need to become aware of reported research so that they may utilize the results in nursing practice.

Format

A research report should be objective, concise and scholarly in spelling, grammar and punctuation. A dictionary and a style manual should be referred to in writing the report. Style manuals have been developed by individual authors such as Campbell and Turabian and by associations such as the American Psychological Association and the Modern Language Association. Additionally, some journals have developed their own style sheets. These are available upon request, or the required format may be found on the journal's front or back cover.

Research reports vary from full, detailed reports to abridged versions for publication. The following format is suggested for preparing a detailed report.

Guidelines for Writing a Research Report

The report is divided into three major parts: I. preliminary materials; II. main body (text) of the report; III. reference materials. Each major part consists of several sections represented in the following outline:

I. Preliminary materials
   A. Title page
   B. Table of contents
   C. List of illustrations (figures)
   D. List of tables
   E. Preface or acknowledgment (if any)

II. Main body (text) of the report

    A. Introduction

        1. Statement of the problem

        2. Review of related literature, including conceptual or theoretical framework

        3. Purpose of the study

        4. Definition of terms

        5. Assumptions of the study

    B. Methodology

        1. Research approach

        2. Study subjects

        3. Techniques for data collection

        4. Procedures

        5. Limitations of the study

    C. Findings

        1. Data are reported and their meaning discussed with no interpretation by the investigator

        2. Tables, graphs, figures are included and discussed in the text

    D. Discussion

        1. Interpretation of findings and conclusions

        2. Comparison of findings with other investigations

        3. Implications for nursing

        4. Recommendations for further study

    E. Summary

        1. Brief restatement of problem

        2. Brief review of procedures, major conclusions, and recommendations

III. Reference materials

    A. Bibliography

    B. Appendix(es) (if any)

    C. Glossary (if any)

Note that the main body (text) of the research report in Appendix E utilizes the research proposal for the study (Appendix D) through the methodology section of the report with few changes.

In the findings section of the report, the data are reported and analyzed objectively with no interpretation by the investigator. Appropriate statistical information is presented and discussed. Each table, graph, or figure used to summarize the data is discussed in the text and should be placed as close as possible to the first reference to it.

In the discussion section of the report, data are interpreted according to the study's purpose and the study results are compared with the results obtained in other studies. The investigator then formulates implications for nursing and recommendations for further research.

In the summary section, the study's most important aspects are presented in a brief restatement of the problem and purpose of the study. A brief review of the data collection procedures and a brief summary of the major conclusions and recommendations are also included.

The bibliography section should list all of the sources used to write the report. A style manual should be used to write this section.

The appendix section includes materials especially designed for the study, such as cover letters or questionnaires. The raw data from the study may be included in this section.

An abstract is a summary of the report. Abstracts vary in length, depending upon their purpose. The information in the summary section of the report can serve as the basis for the abstract.

Application of Research Findings to Nursing Practice

The ultimate aim of conducting research into the practice and profession of nursing, and communicating the results, is to use the knowledge for the improvement of patient care as well as the nursing profession. Nursing research has become a valued activity as nursing strives to identify and construct its scientific knowledge base. In reality, however, there exists a cultural lag between this research knowledge and its application: "A major gap in nursing is translating significant research findings into practice and education." [1]

Ketefian's investigation, for example, asked whether nursing research had an important impact on nursing practice. She determined the extent to which a series of research findings on the mode of temperature determination were being utilized by nursing practitioners. Her conclusion demonstrated this major gap between knowledge and practice:

A clear picture emerged: The practitioner either was totally unaware of the research literature relative to her practice, or, if she was aware of it, was unable to relate to it or utilize it. [2]

The 1970 report of the National Commission for the Study of Nursing and Nursing Education encouraged

the immediate establishment of a national clearinghouse for nursing research to collect, catalogue, and distribute information on investigations completed or in progress. In the case of nursing, with its profound influence on the delivery of optimum health care, we must be concerned that research findings are translated with speed into application and changed practice. [3]

Krueger et al. (1978) also describe the need for a systematic analysis of research studies: "Nursing research must be made accessible by systematic identification, evaluation, and collation of generalizations." [4] These authors assert that this is the responsibility, primarily, of experts in nursing

1. Faye Abdellah, "Overview of Nursing Research, 1955–1968, Part 3," *Nursing Research* 19 (May–June 1970):245.
2. Shaké Ketefian, "Application Of Selected Research Findings into Nursing Practice: A Pilot Study," *Nursing Research* 24 (March–April 1975):91.
3. National Commission for the Study of Nursing and Nursing Education, *An Abstract for Action* (New York: McGraw-Hill, 1970), p. 86.
4. Janelle Krueger, Allen Nelson and Mary Opal Wolanin, *Nursing Research* (Germantown: Aspen Systems Corporation, 1978), p. 337.

practice and research—not the individual nurse—and that the results should be made available through published indices and nursing journals.

Critical Evaluation of Research Reports

As research continues to be an integral and valued part of nursing, leaders in the profession are strongly recommending that research principles and techniques be included in all areas of nursing education. Primarily, nurses should be able to critically review and evaluate nursing studies to differentiate between acceptable and unacceptable research, and to begin to test the results in practice.

Competent evaluation of a research study requires a knowledge of the research process. We have developed general guidelines, utilizing the steps in the research process (Appendix H). These should help you to conduct a systematic evaluation of a research study.

In summary, writing the research report to communicate the study's results and share knowledge is the final step in the research process. The development of a scientific knowledge base through a systematic analysis of research studies is of paramount importance to the nursing profession. The application of this scientific knowledge to the practice setting is the basic goal of nursing research. Each nurse must assume responsibility for critical evaluation of research studies in order to test the ideas in practice, and assist in the development of a scientific knowledge base for nursing.

A Note on Publication

If you decide to write an article for a professional journal based on your research, it is advisable to look over current publications in the area of your study to see where it will have the best chances of being accepted. You should then write a query letter to the editor of the publication to which you would like to submit your article. This letter should include a brief statement of your own background relevant to your article, a brief description of the article you plan to write, and an outline of the article, if possible. You should also request publication guidelines in your letter.

While it is permissible to submit query letters to several publication editors at the same time, the manuscript for the final article should be submitted to only one publication at a time.

A final word: do not become discouraged if your first query letter fails to elicit a positive response. Keep on trying!

The following application activities are designed to help you evaluate your understanding of principles and procedures related to this material.

Application Activities

I. Application of Research Findings to Nursing Practice
1. Discuss the major advantages and disadvantages that you see in the recommendations to identify, evaluate, collate, and publish the findings of nursing research studies.
2. Who should assume the responsibility for implementing this recommendation? Why?
II. Critical Evaluation of Research Reports
1. Use the criteria in the *Guidelines for Evaluating a Research Report* provided in Appendix H to evaluate the research report reprinted in Appendix A. You may want to use the suggested method for estimating the general level of acceptability of the study—being very careful in your interpretation of the percentage—and compare your estimate with your classmates.
2. Use these same *Guidelines* to evaluate a published research study which uses the descriptive research approach.

Bibliography and Suggested Readings

Abdellah, Faye, "Overview of Nursing Research, 1955–1968, Part 3," *Nursing Research* 19 (May–June 1970):239–252.

Fleming, Juanita and Hayter, Jean, "Reading Research Reports Critically," *Nursing Outlook* 22 (March 1974): 172–175.

Gay, L. R. *Educational Research: Competencies for Analysis and Application.* Columbus: Charles E. Merrill Publishing Co., 1976.

Ketefian, Shaké, "Application of Selected Research Findings into Nursing Practice: A Pilot Study," *Nursing Research* 24 (March–April 1975):89–92.

Krueger, J., Nelson, A. and Wolanin, M. *Nursing Research.* Germantown: Aspen Systems Corp., 1978.

National Commission for the Study of Nursing and Nursing Education. *An Abstract For Action.* New York: McGraw-Hill, 1970.

Notter, Lucille. *Essentials of Nursing Research,* 2nd ed. New York: Springer Publishing Co., 1978.

Van Dalen, Deobold. *Understanding Educational Research.* New York: McGraw-Hill, 1973.

Verhonick, Phyllis and Seaman, Catherine. *Research Methods for Undergraduate Students in Nursing.* New York: Appleton-Century-Crofts, 1978.

Wechsler, H. and Kibrick, A. *Explorations in Nursing Research.* New York: Human Sciences Press, 1979.

Part 3

Data Collection Methods for the Research Process

The material in Part 3 is designed to provide you with the principles and techniques for these three major research approaches to data collection:
  Chapter 7: Historical Research Approach
  Chapter 8: Descriptive Research Approach
  Chapter 9: Experimental Research Approach

7

Historical
Research Approach

THE material in this chapter is designed to provide you with the basic principles and methods of the historical research approach.

Nursing is both a very young profession and a very old one. Even before Greek and Roman soldiers were carried home on their shields—sometimes dead and sometimes wounded—someone has always been charged with the care of the ill or injured.

Before 1859 and the Crimean War, nurses of either sex were often camp followers, prostitutes, and thieves. Florence Nightingale's heroic ministrations to the sick and wounded British soldiers, and her devotion to duty, helped to raise nursing to the respectability it enjoys today. However, this respectability did not come about simply as a result of Nightingale's work. Many more subtle battles have been fought against those individuals who have deeply resented the rapid changing of the traditional nursing role.

We do not wish to chronicle Nightingale's life or those of any other heroic characters of nursing. This brief introduction to the founding of modern nursing is intended to set the scene for an examination of the techniques of historical research.

The Nature of Historical Research

Historical research deals with what has happened in the past and how those happenings affect the present. No professional group can truly be said to be more in the forefront of world history than nursing. By its very nature, nursing is always where the action is. Nurses have been active in all areas of the world both in times of conflict and in times of peace, yet nursing history has tended to center around a few semimythologized individuals.

The lives and times of these individuals are important to nursing, but historical research is more than the discovery and adulation of famous individuals. Historical research covers all people. Historians piece together the lives of less well known and less controversial individuals to get a picture of the actual lives and times of an era. The historian uses these data to determine the impact of history on the present and occasionally tries to predict the future based on this knowledge.

Methodology

Essentially, the historian follows the same kind of research format as any other researcher. First, the problem to be investigated must be selected and formulated within the context of existing knowledge and theory. For a historical research study, a hypothesis may be tested. Like any other researcher, the historical researcher must be particularly careful in gathering, interpreting and drawing conclusions based on the data. Historical research lends itself to the acceptance of evidence that is difficult to verify; the careful researcher must do the utmost to corroborate data and to demonstrate their validity and reliability.

Secondary Data Sources

There are a number of data sources available to the historical researcher; they fall into two categories: secondary and primary. Secondary resources are the least trustworthy and are basically of two types: (1) interpretations by someone else on documented data, and (2) hearsay.

Interpretations

Use of interpretations by someone else on documented data is fraught with perils. The historical researcher depends on another person's private frame of reference for information. This means that their interpretations may or may not be totally correct. Just as a television commercial can tell you that almost fifty percent of the people polled preferred "one product over another product" (leaving unstated the fact that more than fifty percent did not prefer this product), so too the historical researcher may choose to emphasize those facts and data which fit his or her hypothesis. This is not good research but it does exist and can lead to further misinterpretation of data. In fact, the further a researcher is from original historical data, the greater the chance of misinterpretation. It is critical that the historical researcher go back to original sources whenever possible. The bibliography and footnotes of the secondary sources often lead to primary sources; then the primary sources can be checked for accuracy of interpretation, and used for gathering additional data. No secondary source, no matter how carefully prepared, can provide a total interpretation of all the data. All historians have to select from a variety of sources and to interpret from them.

Hearsay

The second, and possibly the most naive, secondary sources are those based on hearsay evidence. Hearsay is simply what someone thinks they heard or, even worse, hearsay is the extension of unproven rumors and gossip. We all know how easy it is to misinterpret and pass along incorrect information. The classic example is the *gossip game*. Here a group of people sit in a circle and one person starts the game by whispering a sentence or phrase to the next person. The message is then passed around the circle until it comes back to the originator. It is always interesting to discover how the message changed along the way. Historical researchers must be extremely careful when dealing with hearsay data. It may be old and valuable or it may totally misrepresent the facts. Every effort must be made to corroborate any piece of hearsay data and to place it into proper historical perspective.

Primary Data Sources

Primary data are of far more value and importance to the historian. These data can be found in many forms and many places.

Oral History

One of the most exciting current historical movements is called oral history. With the advent of modern electronic devices such as the tape recorder, it is possible to record the remembrances of older members of the professional community thus providing records of what took place in past periods of time and in specific places. These older persons are invaluable as resources and, as they die, their information is lost forever.

Essentially, the oral historian transcribes the tapes and the conversations are reproduced in writing. Much of these data must be carefully screened but they do provide an important primary history source.

The oral historian should plan a list of questions for the interviewee to help start the conversation off and to stay on the subject. The historian should also get permission to reproduce this information. Many things may be said off the record but this is of no value to the historian. Only evidence for the record can be utilized.

Published Sources

Published sources are quite valuable for the historical researcher. There is an increasing trend to put old newspapers, journals, magazines, and other published material on one of the various microform sources. This means that the historical researcher is not obligated to travel great distances to get to the few remaining copies of the material. Rather, a microfilm copy can be ordered from the producer and reviewed by utilizing microform readers, which are readily available in most college and university libraries and in an increasing number of public libraries. The listing of microforms available can be found in *Microforms in Print*.

Other published sources available are the actual documents themselves. Many items of interest to nurses and nursing can be found in popular literature; early items are indexed in *Poole's Index* and the *Readers' Guide to Periodical Literature*. Neither of these may reflect a complete listing but will aid in the library search.

Government documents are an excellent source for the historical researcher. Our government has compiled enormous quantities of official records and documents. In addition to the federal government, state and local governments also abound with records. Much source data has been lost over the years as county courthouses and other document repositories have burned accidentally, yet many other promising avenues of research are open to the person who is not afraid of the dust and grime usually found in these seldom used sources.

Diaries

Diaries are an invaluable source of documentation. These are often handed down from generation to generation in a family; the researcher must locate families who still have these documents in their possession and are willing to share their intimate contents. This research requires judicious questioning and a substantial amount of very careful exploration.

Historical Societies

Often, there will be a local historical group that a researcher can contact. These groups are justifiably proud of their community's history, and can provide access to many documents and to individuals with specific knowledge. All of this can be invaluable to an outside researcher.

Official Minutes

Obviously, the availability of minutes and records of meetings is important. It is wise to remember, however, that minutes of meetings usually reflect an abridged version of what really happened. Acrimonious debate or nonvoted issues often are not shown in minutes. Remember, each legislator has the privilege of editing what he or she has said on the floor of the House or Senate before such speeches are finally placed in the Congressional Record. Thus, the speeches we read are not necessarily verbatim reports of what was actually said.

Audio and Video Recordings

Current technology has made a great deal of audio and video source material available. Records, tape and wire recordings, film and video tapes all may provide invaluable historical insight. Much of this material may be rare and hard to obtain. Locating appropriate sources can be a tedious, yet fascinating job.

Eyewitnesses

Eyewitness accounts are always useful. Written eyewitness accounts may be found in newspapers, as oral history, or in diaries. It is crucial that eyewitness accounts receive corroboration from other sources, because such accounts may report only a small part of the whole.

Pictorial Sources

Photographs and other pictorial sources, such as sketches, are extremely valuable items. The old Chinese saying that "One picture is worth a thousand words" can be very true.

Certainly Mathew Brady and other photographers of the Civil War provided visual portraits of times and places that only could be imagined if we had nothing more than the written documents. Again, even as personal diaries are rich resources, so are family picture albums. They can be used to find out a great deal about the history of a group of people in any locality.

Other Print Sources

Other valid source materials for historical research might be old telephone books and directories, catalogues of local businesses and national concerns, and accounting books and bank records.

Physical Evidence

Do not ignore physical evidence of change throughout the years. For example, there have been many alterations in the various types of equipment used by nurses. Many of the products of technical change which have been added to the repertoire of nursing can be used as source materials for historical research.

Validity and Reliability

In all cases, the historical researcher must question the reliability and validity of sources by applying both internal and external criticism to the written document. External criticism deals with the validity of the document—is it really what it purports to be? Internal criticism deals with the reliability or accuracy of the information. Some of the questions that should be asked include: Is this document consistent with other documents written by this person? Does it have the same style? Does the style match the style of the time? Are spelling and handwriting consistent with the time? Is what the document says true? Remember, it is very

easy to fool a naive researcher—documents can be manufactured. Caution is the watchword when dealing with
historical material.

In this chapter we discussed the techniques and principles of historical research. Discovering the past through
careful documentation can provide many important insights
into the present.

Application Activities

Read the historical research proposal in Appendix B. Notice how
the researcher carefully delineates her topic and provides careful
checks on the validity and reliability of the data sources to provide accurate data interpretation. Note also how the researcher
focuses on primary sources, and defends her uses of such sources,
while being aware of the potential hazards of historical research.

Bibliography and Suggested Readings

Austen, Anne L. *History of Nursing Sourcebook*. New York:
G. P. Putnam's Sons, 1957.

Benjamin, Jules R. *A Student's Guide to History*. New York:
St. Martin's Press, 1975.

Christy, T. E. "The Methodology of Historical Research,"
Nursing Research 24 (May–June 1975):189–192.

Clark, G. Kitson. *Guide for Research Students Working on
Historical Subjects*. 2nd ed. London: Cambridge University Press, 1969.

Dock, Lavina L. *A History of Nursing*. New York: G. P.
Putnam's Sons, 1912.

Dock, Lavina L., Stewart, Isabel. *A Short History of Nursing*.
New York: G. P. Putnam's Sons, 1920.

Roberts, Mary M. *American Nursing: History and Interpretation*. New York: Macmillan Co., 1954.

8

Descriptive Research Approach

THE material in this chapter is designed to acquaint you with the descriptive research approach—also termed survey research—and the techniques and tools most frequently used to gather data needed to study present conditions.

The Nature of Descriptive Research

The descriptive research approach is present oriented in that it describes what is as it now exists. The term is not completely appropriate, since description is also involved in the other two approaches. Historical research describes the past, and experimental research describes what happens to selected variables in predicting what will be as other variables are manipulated by the investigator. The term is used here to refer to research questions and problems based in the present state of affairs or real world settings, that have implications for generating new knowledge beyond the study's specific subjects or elements.

Descriptive Research Techniques

The techniques for gathering data about present conditions are intended to provide information that is both objective and quantifiable, that is, measurable. The techniques most often used to study present conditions, which can be used to study contrasts (differences), comparisons (likenesses) and relationships, include:

1. Questionnaires and interviews
2. Rating scales
3. Content analysis
4. Use of available data
5. Observation
6. Participant observation
7. Unobtrusive measures
8. Nonwritten records
9. Case studies
10. Psychological and projective tests
11. Sociometrics
12. Delphi technique
13. Electric or mechanical devices

Each of these techniques will be discussed in greater detail on the following pages.

Questionnaires and Interviews

The term *survey research* is often used to refer to the collection of data about present conditions directly from the study subjects. The most common techniques for survey research are the questionnaire and the interview.

The term *questionnaire* refers to a paper and pencil instrument completed by the study subjects themselves. In survey research, the questionnaire is usually mailed to the respondents, although it might be administered face to face. An *opinionnaire* is a questionnaire designed to elicit the subjects' opinions. The term *interview* refers to verbal questioning of respondents by the investigator in order to collect data. The interview may be conducted either face-to-face or by telephone.

Nursing researchers have developed numerous survey instruments—primarily questionnaires—over the years. The repondents may be nurses, patients, patients' relatives, doctors, or any one of many alternatives. These survey instruments have been designed to examine attitudes, opinions, feelings and facts concerning certain areas of nursing. Such instruments can accurately reflect these opinions, feelings and facts only if they are well developed, well administered, and carefully interpreted.

LONGITUDINAL STUDIES   Occasionally, investigators with long term interests and long term financing will use the same measuring instrument again and again to determine responses on a topic and to pinpoint trends and issues. Such studies are designed to collect data from the same people at regularly stated intervals, ranging from a few days apart to weeks, months or even years. These are known as *longitudinal studies*.

CROSS-SECTIONAL STUDIES   The vast majority of surveys, however, are one time *cross-sectional studies*. That is, they study certain aspects of responses at a certain point in time and are seldom, if ever, conducted again. This is unfortunate because it leads to the proliferation of data gathering instruments, some of which may not be very good. In addition, the lack of repeated measures over time precludes the analysis of trends about various issues.

Surveys can be used to gather information from a representative sample of a population. The researcher can specify the location of the population, such as all patients admitted to the emergency room of XYZ Hospital, or only those patients admitted to the emergency room between the hours of noon to midnight. Such specificity allows for the use of probability sampling techniques and, with good statistical analysis, generalizations can be drawn about the whole population. As discussed in Chapter 4, when developing a research proposal, care must be taken to insure an accurate description of the target population as well as the sample. Whether the population be 24- to 27-year-old postpartum mothers with female infants, or any other of an infinitely large number of combinations, the best research is very specific about who will be surveyed.

With these ideas in mind, we will now describe the steps in designing and carrying out survey research by questionnaires.

Questionnaires: Development and Administration

First, as in the case of any research study, an appropriate research question or problem must be established. The problem statement and the purpose of the study should guide the selection of an appropriate survey research design, and the choice of a measuring instrument, such as a questionnaire. We have already discussed the advantages of using an existing instrument that meets the criteria of validity, reliability, and usability in Chapter 4. The following principles apply to self-developed questionnaires constructed by the investigator for a specific study.

In constructing a questionnaire, care must be exercised so that the items will allow the respondents to provide the information that relates to the study problem and to the purpose of the study. The theoretical or conceptual framework should provide the rationale for the development of the questionnaire.

Questionnaires are constructed to be either open-ended or closed. Open-ended questionnaires allow the respondents a variety of ways to answer questions, and permit the researcher to make inferences from the responses to the questions. Closed questionnaires allow for certain structured answers, that is, "yes," or "no," or a limited selection of choices. Since most survey researchers want to speed the coding of data and eliminate ambiguity, they will most frequently opt for a closed questionnaire.

The questionnaire must be very clear and unambiguous. We all assume that people understand what we are talking about and we usually have a common frame of reference when talking to someone. The naive respondent may not have the same frame of reference as the researcher. The old saying, "Do you still beat your wife?" is a good example of the ambiguity of our language. Similarly, any question that can have multiple interpretations should be avoided.

The wording of questions should be concise. Avoid asking a question using a lot of words when a few will do. Respondents who do not understand because of vocabulary differences will not give accurate or valid answers. At the same time, respect the respondent's intelligence. This means walking a fine line. The more confusion or mistrust caused by the instrument, the less chance there will be that the respondent will return the questionnaire.

Keep the instrument as simple and short as possible. No one wants to face a long, involved questionnaire. There is something very threatening about a many-paged instrument with a multiplicity of choices. The shorter the instrument (within reason) the more likely it is to be returned and completed. Be sure to put relatively simple questions at the beginning of the instrument. This allows the respondent to succeed and be reinforced to continue.

Cross-check questions should be provided in order to be sure that the respondent is answering consistently. Rewording and asking the same question is a good way to provide this insurance, but questions should be sufficiently separated so that the subject will not see through this relatively transparent technique.

Finally, careful development of the instructions for the respondent involves a clear statement of what you want the respondent to do. Validity and reliability must be determined by using any one of the techniques described in Chapter 4. The authors strongly recommend that a pretest of the questionnaire be conducted in order to correct any problem with the questionnaire prior to administering it to the study subjects.

Researchers should probably spend more time formulating their questionnaires than they do analyzing their research data. Well-constructed questionnaires allow for relatively easy interpretations and analyses. Poorly developed questionnaires may cost even more in time and effort, and will prevent the investigator from achieving the purpose of the study.

Mailed questionnaires are responded to in much larger numbers if a self-addressed, stamped envelope is included with each questionnaire. Most people are willing to respond, but are unwilling to subsidize the researcher. If a follow-up letter is sent it may be wise to send yet another self-addressed, stamped envelope and questionnaire. Granted, this may add to the researcher's expenditures, but all research should be planned out to include the total cost of all items.

Cover letters are important and should include the following items:

1. the name of the researcher
2. the address of the researcher
3. the purpose of the study
4. the approximate length of time required to fill out the questionnaire
5. a statement safeguarding the confidentiality of responses
6. any other information the researcher feels is important

For an example of a cover letter see the one reprinted in Appendix C.

When using a mailed questionnaire, the investigator allows a specified amount of time to elapse after the survey instrument has been mailed, and determines an acceptable percentage of responses to be obtained. This is necessary because there are many reasons for nonresponses to any survey, especially if the survey instrument is mailed. Any investigator who expects to wait until a one hundred percent response is obtained will probably never draw any conclusions from the study!

Interviews

In face-to-face administration of a questionnaire, the principles of interviewing should be followed. These are discussed in the following section.

There are two basic kinds of interviewing techniques: the structured and the unstructured. In the *structured interview,* the interviewer has a list of prepared questions that the researcher believes will provide a format for the respondent's answers concerning the researcher's project. For example:

1. How friendly do the nurses in ZZZ Hospital seem to be?
2. Why do you answer as you do? (and so forth)

Here we see that the interviewer guides the respondent to determine what information is to be elicited and records the answers.

An *unstructured interview* is more like a conversation. Here the researcher has a general framework of questions to elicit answers concerning the information sought, but seizes upon the respondent's answers to enlarge upon the topic and to ask additional questions. The topics flow from the conversation's progress, and there is no set pattern or ordering of the categories which the researcher is exploring. Unstructured interviews take more time than structured interviews, and force the researcher to search the record of responses to categorize and organize the data elicited.

It is always the responsibility of the investigator to provide adequate training for the interviewers who may be assisting in the collection of the study data. Face-to-face interviewers must be selected to represent a minimum threat to the respondent. Certain styles of dress and manners may be appropriate in one setting and not in another. Each interviewer must gain rapport and trust with the respondent— first impressions are extremely important. Interviewers should be trained to be as neutral as possible when eliciting answers to the survey instrument. Many people will give the answer that they believe the interviewer wants to hear and not what they really believe. Interviewers who encourage such responses overtly or unconsciously cannot gather valid data.

A pilot or preliminary study is extremely valuable as a part of the training process. Debriefing after a few interviews allows the interviewers to point out flaws not initially discovered in the interview schedules and coding sheets. It also provides for a check on interviewing techniques.

Remember, too, that the interviewer will be doing two separate things during the course of the interview. First, the questions or statements must be given to the respondent and the appropriate response elicited. Second, the interviewer will be marking a coded response sheet or recording what the respondent says. Obviously, the statements on the response sheet must be organized carefully so that the interviewer can perform these tasks with a minimum of problems. If it is physically difficult to code the responses, the chances for errors increase significantly.

It is usually easier to gain interviews if the interviewers have official sanction. For example, when planning to interview members of a community, contacting local city officials is often helpful. Frequently they will be willing to provide a letter, badge or other symbol of official recognition. This can provide much easier access to study subjects by enhancing the trust of the respondents. It is well to remember that in a small community news travels rapidly. If the interviewing techniques are not pleasing, potential respondents may reject the interviewers based on what they have heard from others in the community.

Telephone interviewers should also be selected with care. Respondents visualize the individual on the other end of the line, so the interviewer should have a pleasing telephone voice and should have practiced using the survey instrument a number of times before actually talking to potential respondents.

It is well to note that people appear to be increasingly resistant to responding to telephone surveys. This may be due to a number of reasons. First, with the increasing popularity of telephone surveys, individuals find that their time is being demanded more frequently. Second, there have been frequent misrepresentations of surveys by telephone solicitors who claim to be conducting a survey but are actually selling a product. Finally, more and more people have come to resent the intrusion of surveys into their privacy.

Respondents should be given an opportunity to receive the results of the study. After being a respondent in any survey, the individual has a vested interest in finding out what came about as a result of the study. The offer to provide a summary of the study's results will often entice individuals who might not otherwise participate or respond. Be sure to keep your word. Failing to provide the promised information is a quick way to ruin future research possibilities both for yourself and others. As the investigator, you have a responsibility for complete honesty to your repsondents and the researchers of the future. People resent being used and many of them want to know what happened as a result of their participation in a study.

Rating Scales

A *rating scale* is a type of data collecting technique that allows the respondents to place their feelings or attitudes on a scale. For example:

How would you rate the nursing care in this hospital?
Very good ——:——:——:——:—— Very poor
please check the appropriate box

The number of response options on rating scales may vary considerably. While five options occur most frequently and this appears to be the minimum acceptable number, six, seven, or eight options can also be presented. The term *Likert Scale* refers to a rating scale in which each statement usually has five possible responses: strongly agree, agree, uncertain, disagree, strongly disagree.

There is a definite advantage in using even number scales. These are called *forced choice* scales. when given an odd number of choices, subjects may respond to the middle choice and thus appear to be neutral, perceiving neither high nor low ratings. If a scale has an even number of options, the subject must respond with a high or low ranking or rating. Given the previous question, the forced choice scale compels the respondent to like or dislike the nursing care.

Very Good ——:——:——:——:——:—— Very poor

If the sample size is small, sometimes adequate statistical analysis cannot be done. This type of scale allows for the collapsing of cells (categories of data), for dichotomization or for bringing cells together in statistically valid groups. Neutral responses might otherwise have to be discarded or divided, giving an unclear picture of the respondents' feelings or attitudes.

The scale might similarly have been written:
The nursing care in this hospital is very good.
VSA SA A D SD VSD

The responses stand for: very strongly agree, strongly agree, agree, disagree, strongly disagree, very strongly disagree. In this instance, the respondent would probably be asked to circle the most appropriate response.

Respondents may be asked to *rank order* their responses from most important to least important. This technique can be very effective. If the rank order list is too long, however, the subjects may have difficulty in keeping the whole list in mind. For example:

Nurses should be capable of participating in research. Below is a list of settings in which nursing research can be carried out. Please rank each in order of importance as a setting for nursing research by placing a "6" by the most important, a "5" by the second most important and so on to number "1" (least important).

( ) hospital
( ) community health center
( ) visiting nurses' association
( ) hospice
( ) day care center
( ) home health agency

A type of rating scale that has had a great deal of interest and success is called the *semantic differential*. This tool is composed of a list of polar adjectives which may describe a setting, an object, a profession, or many other variables.

For example, if we want to determine how people from different cultural and ethnic groups and backgrounds perceive hospitals, we might construct the following:

Below is a list of words that describe a hospital. Please place a check mark in the space that best shows how you feel about hospitals. Be sure to place a check on each line.

Hospitals

Good	—:	—:	—:	—:	—:	—:	—	Bad
Busy	—:	—:	—:	—:	—:	—:	—	Quiet
Warm	—:	—:	—:	—:	—:	—:	—	Cold
Clean	—:	—:	—:	—:	—:	—:	—	Dirty

Various analytical techniques can be applied to the items in a *semantic differential scale* to determine if different subjects perceive the hospital setting in different ways.

Multiple choice questions have long been a staple for examinations. They may also be used for eliciting research data. For example:

Place a circle around the letter of the response that most accurately reflects your point of view about the following items.
1. People have strong feelings about a national health care program. Which of the following statements best represents your attitude toward national health care?
   a. National health care will cost too much to be practical and should be avoided.
   b. National health care is the only way to provide adequate health care for all of the people.
   c. National health care should be limited to catastrophic illnesses.
   d. National health care would subvert our free enterprise system.

Note that in this instance respondents may not agree with any of the choices. Care must be exercised in developing this kind of instrument so that experimenter bias does not creep in through the use of slanted questions.

Content Analysis

Up to this point, we have been discussing closed or structured measuring instruments: instruments that allow the respondents few or no alternatives in their responses. Frequently— as you probably have experienced—there is a feeling or response of "yes, but. . . ." The respondents would like to qualify their answers by fleshing out or providing reasons for their answers. Open-ended measuring instruments allow respondents to explain why they respond in a particular manner. For example:

> Do you believe that the hospital staff should be differentiated by the color of their uniforms? Blue for RNs, Green for aides, Yellow for LPNs, etc.? Please explain your answer.

This type of instrument lends itself to *content analysis*. The researcher examines the responses to determine the most frequently cited reasons, compares adjective usage between different groups, or utilizes one of a large number of potential analytical techniques. Obviously, with large samples and many responses, the technique becomes extremely tedious. Careful analysis of the content of the responses can reveal a great deal about the respondents, however, that might otherwise be lost if closed or structured measuring instruments were used.

Use of Available Data

Over the years, there has been an increasing number of nursing studies. These studies have created a large pool of *available data*. Studies that give complete reports of the number of respondents and their responses can be reanalyzed using other statistical tools to determine if the conclusions were as accurate as the original researcher reported. These tools are often more sophisticated due to technological advances than those available to the original researcher. Further, com-

parisons and contrasts can be made between past study responses and current study responses. For example, there has
been a renewed interest in the study of sociobiology that is
causing a great deal of controversy at present. Reanalysis of
existing data from sociobiological studies done at the turn
of the century might well be a valid research project at this
time. Many such data are open to reinterpretation based on
current knowledge and techniques.

Other available data sources include the reports of the
large number of specialized statistical gathering organizations, census tract reports, licensing bureau reports, and the
reports of other organizations that gather and report data
about people or groups of people. For example, a college
placement service might have information about the type
and level of employment held by the graduates of a certain
program. This might lead to conclusions about the success
of an institution in educating its students.

Observation

When the researcher is concerned with motives, habits, styles
of thinking, and other attributes that may be difficult to
elicit by the use of survey instruments, there are a number
of observational techniques which lend themselves to description and analysis of behavior.

The structured check list is one technique used for
observation. What happens and how often it happens is
recorded to determine the frequency of certain events or
activities. For example, a study's purpose may be to determine if laryngectomy patients behave differently postopera-
tively as a result of structured preoperative teaching about
their surgery as opposed to a different kind of instruction.
The researcher creates a check list of significant behavioral
activities to record the postoperative behaviors of the patients
being observed in the study. The researcher then determines
the frequency of occurrences and tallies the results. This provides the foundation for interpretations and conclusions on

the effect of structured preoperative teaching on the post-operative behavior of laryngectomy patients.

Observation research often requires that several observers be used. This means that there is a potential for differences of observations among the observers. Consequently, the researcher must be extremely careful to train the observers by providing common experiences so that observer reliability can be established. Given the example of the laryngectomy patient study, observers could be shown films or videotapes of patients performing a range of behaviors. The observers would then mark the designated activities on their observation check list and their perception could be checked by the researcher. By providing a number of training sessions of this nature, observer reliability could be determined.

Participant Observation

There can be times when the researcher may not be able to formulate specific checklists of activities to be observed. The researcher must then catalogue all activities, or as many as possible, and then determine which activities are significant and which are trivial. This essentially is the technique used by social anthropologists. The social anthropological researcher often becomes a participant as well as an observer and attempts to elicit usable data by unstructured interviews and observations.

For example, there are many ways to examine beliefs about diseases and how to effect cures of these diseases. There are also many groups of people in the developed as well as the nondeveloped countries who practice various kinds of folk medicine to achieve cures. Disease etiology and classification are important to a nurse who is attempting to communicate with a patient. How the illness is perceived and is described by the patient is a critical area for research.

Examples of such participant observation studies might include: studying disease classifications among Spanish speaking migrant workers, the root medicine still practiced in many areas of the rural South, the continuation of various healing activities of American Indian groups, or the use of health foods and herbs in the population at large.

It is the responsibility of the participant observer to make frequent and valid notes. Many observers are forced by time considerations to develop a kind of shorthand to jot down observations made on the spot. Then, at a later time, a full description of the event or events is written down. Common sense dictates that such observations be recorded in full as soon as possible in order to preclude forgetting what those scribbles really meant.

The researcher who uses participant observation is limited as to the number of individuals with whom contacts can be made. Frequently, first contacts may be with marginal individuals who need social contacts and/or approval, and whose information may be unreliable. Therefore, the researcher must be careful that the data gathered are accurate and valid. A study of witchcraft beliefs might be extremely difficult to document, for example, because of the fear of the respondents that they might be accused of witchcraft. They may believe they would become victims of witchcraft if they tell of known witches. Rapport and trust are crucial if the researcher is to obtain any kind of valid information.

Unobtrusive measures

There has been an increasing number of studies using *unobtrusive measures* over the years. The researcher decides what needs to be measured and then determines how to measure it without direct intervention. A time-honored way to measure the most popular exhibits in a museum would be to determine the dirtiest display cases at the end of a day; this is done on the assumption that the more people who lean on a display case the dirtier it will be. Over a period of time, certain exhibits would show the most consistent usage.[1]

---

1. Eugene Webb et al. *Unobtrusive Measures: Non-Reactive Research in the Social Sciences* (Chicago: Rand McNally and Company, 1965), pp. 45–46.

Similarly, counting the cigarette butts in ashtrays in the expectant fathers' waiting room in the maternity ward might provide information if a researcher wanted to determine whether repeated warnings about cigarette smoking and health hazards have had any effect. Anxiety levels could be measured by the wear and tear on magazines placed in waiting rooms. Perhaps more stress is exhibited in the office of a dentist than in the waiting room of a maternity ward. It might be fun to find out!

Nonwritten Records

There are a number of techniques available that preserve the activities of the subjects in an enduring format. In the past, still photographs and pictures were used frequently to analyze the behavior, beliefs, dress and activities of individuals and groups. With the advent of motion pictures and sound motion pictures, far more details could be captured. Today, these techniques as well as the technology of video and audio tapes can provide long-lasting records for future use and study.

Case Studies

Case studies might be considered a particular methodology within the descriptive research technique. Social anthropologists have long been concerned with rather large groups of individuals, especially those sharing a common culture or background. In the *case study method,* a general population sharing a common background is identified but the researcher works with a limited number of individuals, ranging from one or two to a larger sample. The researcher then carefully observes and documents all of the activities, contacts and other salient actions of the individual(s).

Using the case study method, a nurse might document the activities of several hospital supervisors to determine if differences in leadership styles existed in the obstetrical service as opposed to the intensive care units.

Psychological and Projective Tests

Frequently, we may want to determine more than surface attitudes about something. Perhaps we are trying to understand why the patient feels as he or she feels. Since it is impossible to look into a person's brain to determine what is happening, inferential instruments must be used. Consistency of responses can indicate a frame of reference, a mind set, or a set of ideas.

Psychiatry and psychology have developed a number of instruments to determine a patient's feelings. These are called *projective tests* because the patient projects a meaning into materials which are essentially ambiguous or meaningless.

We have all heard of the Rorschach (Ink Blot) Test. Here an individual is asked to look at a standard series of abstract forms (ink blots), some of which are black and white, some multicolored, and asked to tell what he or she sees. Since the forms are random in shape, the subject must project or put meaning into them from his or her own beliefs or ideas. By presenting a series of these items, the researcher can draw conclusions about the subject's state of mind.

The Thematic Apperception Test (TAT) is also frequently used to determine feelings and ideas. In this test, subjects are shown pictures of people in ambiguous situations and asked to describe what is happening. Again, the subject must project his or her own feelings into the situations; the researcher can then draw conclusions about the individual.

Projective tests can be very helpful, but the researcher must be careful to interpret the responses carefully. The very nature of the devices can lead to misunderstanding and misinterpretations. Much planning and training is necessary before these devices can be put into use by a researcher.

As discussed in Chapter 4, the authors strongly suggest that you go to as many sources as possible to determine if a pre-existing measuring instrument is available. Frequently, an appropriate instrument is available with reliability and validity already established. A few hours of library search with such resources as *Mental Measurements Yearbook* or *Tests in Print* may well preclude several weeks of development time.

Sociometrics

Sometimes the researcher wants to determine the social interaction and patterns of leadership roles in a group. This can be determined by the use of sociometric techniques. Essentially, the researcher structures a questionnaire to determine the most desirable, or the most favorably perceived individuals, in a group.

Questions to determine sociometrics might include:

1. Who is the best nurse on the unit?
2. Which nurses are the most effective? Name three.
3. Which three nurses do you like working with the best?

After eliciting responses to several questions, the researcher can determine the social makeup of the group in a variety of ways.

You may want to develop a sociogram to diagram the responses (see page 144).

You may want to develop a social matrix showing the responses in tabular form.

Table 8–1 Social Matrix

SELECTEE	SELECTOR					
	LEE	CLAIRE	EVELYN	LOU	JOE	BOBBIE
Lee	—	X	X		X	X
Claire	X	—		X		
Evelyn		X	—			
Lou			X	—	X	X
Joe	X			X	—	X
Bobbie	X	X	X	X	X	—

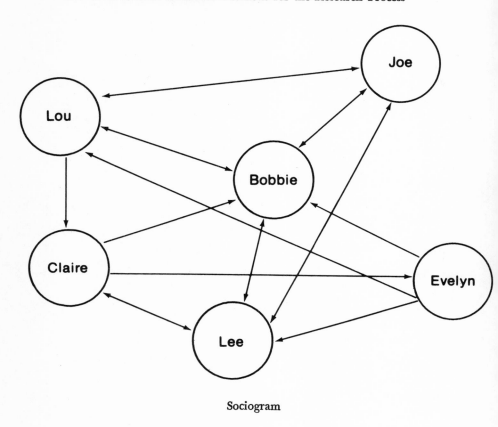

Sociogram

This technique can provide some very important information about the group's informal structure, who the informal leaders are, and where the power really lies within the group's structure.

Delphi Technique

One survey technique that has been very popular in the past few years is the Delphi Technique. Named after the famous Greek Oracle at Delphi, the process attempts to predict what will be important to the surveyed group in the future.

Essentially, the Delphi Technique consists of identifying a group of experts or persons concerned with a certain

area or program. Their concerns about their area or program are elicited and ranked. Once a total list of concerns
has been acquired, it is given to the experts and they are
asked to rate them in importance.

The responses are again tallied by the researcher and
sent back to the same panel with the totals of responses
given. The panel members are then asked to rerank their
responses on the basis of the total responses and their peer's
evaluations. The researcher can then focus on those items
considered the most important by the experts.

For example, we might use the Delphi Technique to
examine nurses' concerns in a community health agency by
sending out the following questions to all, or a sample, of
the staff nurses:

We are attempting to determine the future goals for
patient care in a community setting. Please list at least
five of your major concerns about nursing service as it
is currently practiced and how it should be practiced
in a community setting.

As you can see, each of the respondents then has an
opportunity to predict the future of nursing care in the
community.

After the first round of responses is returned, the researcher lists each comment—with similar comments organized into a single topic—and a questionnaire is developed.
The same respondents are used in all rounds of questioning
so that a letter such as the following might be sent to the
initial respondents:

Several weeks ago you were asked to list your major
concerns about the patient care in your community.
As a result of your responses, and those of your peers,
we have been able to develop the following list of concerns. We would now like you to rate these concerns
on a scale of one to five with one being of little importance and five being of great importance.
1. Patient loads are too large for adequate care to be
given.   1 2 3 4 5

2. Patients are unable to get additional care from other community agencies.   1   2   3   4   5

After the subjects respond to this questionnaire, the researcher then calculates how each response was evaluated by determining the percentages of the total responses in each category. For instance, the group sampled on the question concerning patient loads might have responded 60% 5's, 20% 4's and 20% 3's. Another survey is then sent to the respondents with a letter that might read like this:

> You and your colleagues have responded to a series of questions concerning nursing care in your community. Each of you was asked to rank a list of questions as to their importance. Based upon your responses, the questions were rated by the percentages in the categories which you see below. Next to the percentages there is another rating scale. Please rate the questions as to their importance, again, based on your own beliefs and your knowledge of your peers' responses.

At this point, the subjects may also be supplied with their own previous responses. The subjects then respond and rate the questions as to their relative importance. The researcher reevaluates the scale and determines which items are now considered the most important by the respondents. The researcher then identifies the main areas of concern and makes recommendations.

The Delphi Technique has the advantage of identifying the group's major concerns and can be used to make recommendations to alleviate these concerns. It also allows an organization to focus on and take direction toward the future.

Electric or Mechanical Devices

By its very nature, nursing research lends itself to the use of highly accurate physiological measurements. There are an increasing number of sophisticated measuring devices (based on technological developments) available to determine physiological responses. Of course, the classical mechanical devices such as the sphygmomanometer and the stethescope have been developed and refined over many years. Many electronic devices, however, such as the electrocardiograph and the electroencephalograph, as well as other instruments, are now available. Note, in the study concerned with the treatment of decubitus ulcers with topical application of insulin (Appendix A), the devices used for physiological measurement consisted simply of waxed paper and graph paper.

As in all research dealing with human subjects, when mechanical or electric devices are used, nurses have the ethical responsibility to obtain informed consent and to explain the purposes of any devices that are used to determine the patients' responses. There is something extremely frightening about being attached to some sort of mechanical or electrical device without knowing the reason for it.

In summary, the descriptive research approach is present oriented as it describes what now exists. The descriptive research approach techniques most often used include: (1) questionnaires and interviews; (2) rating scales; (3) content analysis; (4) use of available data; (5) observation; (6) participant observation; (7) unobtrusive measures; (8) nonwritten records; (9) case studies; (10) psychological and projective techniques; (11) sociometrics; (12) Delphi technique; and (13) electric or mechanical devices.

In each case, the techniques and instruments must be carefully selected and evaluated to determine their appropriateness for collecting the study data. Researchers must exercise a great deal of caution in developing appropriate instruments for their research. Careful attention must be paid to the fundamental questions of validity, reliability and usability, as well as to time and cost constraints. In order to apply the principles presented, you should complete the application activities listed below.

Application Activities

1. Examine your research problem carefully. Does it require an electric or mechanical measurement? If so, describe the device(s) that you can use.

2. If you are using a survey instrument, is there an electric or mechanical device that might be used in conjunction to validate respondents' answers?
3. Look in a nursing journal that publishes research studies. Examine and list the techniques for gathering data used by the researchers in at least three issues of the same journal. Is any one technique used more frequently than others?
4. Read the article "An Experience in Participant Observation" by Bettie S. Jackson listed in the Bibliography and Suggested Readings for this chapter. Discuss the conflict between the nurse as observer and the nurse as the provider of nursing care.

Bibliography and Suggested Readings

Agnew, Neil McK.; Pyke, Sandraw. *The Science Game.* 2nd ed. Englewood Cliffs, N.J.: Prentice-Hall, 1978.

Anastasi, Anne. *Psychological Testing.* 4th ed. New York: Macmillan Co., 1976.

Babbie, E. *Survey Research Methods.* Belmont, Calif.: Wadsworth Publishing Co., 1973.

Cromwell, Leslie et al. *Biomedical Instrumentation and Measurements.* Englewood Cliffs, N.J.: Prentice-Hall, 1973.

Forcese, Dennis; Richer, Stephen. *Social Research Methods.* Englewood Cliffs, N.J.: Prentice-Hall, 1973.

Geddes, Leslie; Baker, L. E. *Principals of Applied Biomedical Instrumentation.* 3rd ed. New York: John Wiley and Sons, 1975.

Gordon, R. L. *Interviewing: Strategy, Techniques and Tactics.* Homewood, Ill.: Dorsey Press, 1975.

Holsti, O. R. *Content Analysis for the Social Sciences and Humanities.* Reading, Mass.: Addison-Wesley, 1969.

Jackson, Bettie S. "An Experience in Participant Observation," *Nursing Outlook,* 23 (September 1975):552–555.

Kerlinger, Fred N. *Foundations of Behavioral Research.* 2nd ed. New York: Holt, Rinehart and Winston, 1973.

Linstone, Harold; Turoff, Murray, eds. *The Delphi Method:*

Techniques and Application. Reading, Mass.: Addison-Wesley, 1975.

Osgood, C. E.; Suci, G. J.; Tannenbaum, P. H. *The Measurement of Meaning.* Urbana, Ill.: University of Illinois Press, 1957.

Pelto, Pertti J. *Anthropological Research: The Structure of Inquiry.* New York: Harper & Row, 1970.

Rosenthal, Robert. *Experimenter Effects in Behavioral Research.* New York: Appleton-Century-Crofts, 1966.

Sackman, Harold. *Delphi Critique: Expert Opinion, Forecasting, and Group Process.* Lexington, Mass.: Lexington Books, 1975.

Van Dalen, Deobold B. *Understanding Educational Research: An Introduction.* 3rd ed. New York: McGraw-Hill, 1973.

Vredevoe, Donna L. "Nursing Research Involving Physiological Mechanisms: Definitions of Variables." *Nursing Research* 21 (January–February 1972):68–72.

Wax, Rosalie H. *Doing Fieldwork: Warnings and Advice.* Chicago: University of Chicago Press, 1971.

Webb, Eugene et al. *Unobtrusive Measures: Nonreactive Research in the Social Sciences.* Chicago: Rand McNally, 1966.

Williamson, John B. et al. *The Research Craft.* Boston: Little, Brown, 1977.

9

Experimental Research Approach

THE material in this chapter is designed to introduce you to some basic principles and methods on the experimental research approach. When researching a nursing problem, we seek solutions that we hope will improve patient care and enhance the quality of life for all people. One of the great problems in seeking solutions to research problems is that we are dealing with human beings who often tend to report a wide variety of feelings, attitudes, or even misunderstandings. Obviously, the researcher wants to control as many factors as possible; this leads to utilizing an experimental approach and to the development of experimental design methodology.

The Nature of Experimental Research

Experimental design is based on the notion of control. Observed instances of an activity may or may not be the cause of a consequence. The experimenter wants to determine if the activity was or was not the cause of the effect observed. For example, parents, teachers, and others admonish, "don't get your feet wet or you'll catch cold." This appears to be a reasonable statement, yet we know that colds are caused by viruses that are transmitted from one person to another. Foot wetting in and of itself will not cause a person to catch a cold. It may make the person uncomfortable, disturb physiological balance and lower resistance to infection but, alone, foot wetting is not the causal factor in colds. Many common sense ideas are rooted in the folklore of cause and effect; the careful researcher designs experiments to verify if, indeed, the cause does bring about the observed effect.

As already mentioned, working with human beings makes experimental research extremely difficult. Controls are difficult to apply, and many techniques used on plants and animals are certainly not open to experimenters who utilize human subjects. We advise you to reexamine the discussion now regarding the protection of human subjects (Appendix F) to fully appreciate the researcher's responsibilities for the protection of human rights.

In nursing research, the investigator may want to vary certain factors that appear to have causal relationships to something else. In the article on the application of topical insulin to decubitus ulcers (Appendix A), the experimenters were concerned with the reduction of decubitus ulcers through the application of insulin. The researchers attempted to control as many factors as possible and, where not possible, to compensate for their potential effects. In the experiment measuring the effect of a constantly moving bed on the respiratory status of immobilized patients (Appendix D), the motion of the bed was hypothesized to affect arterial blood gas values but no statistically significant difference was observed.

It is worthwhile, again, to mention the idea of statistical significance. A desired level of outcome is established prior to carrying out the research plan. Frequently the result is not statistically significant and the researcher goes away feeling that the research has been for naught. Nothing could be farther from the truth. Research studies that yield no statistical significance, if carefully planned and executed are just as valid as studies that yield statistically significant differences. There are probably several reasons why researchers have the idea that their research is not acceptable if no statistically significant difference is found. First, most researchers want to reject the null hypothesis. They believe the experimental approach they are using is better than some other approach. Researchers often have a vested interest in the success of their experiments. They find it terribly disappointing to discover that their great ideas did not work out as expected.

Second, as we review the literature, we quickly discover

that research journals tend to report studies with highly significant results. This attitude has come about over the years and is potentially damaging to the research process. Editors of some journals will report only those studies that are highly significant and do not publish equally valid studies that show no statistically significant differences.

Third, we must remember that statistics developed outside of the area of human subject research. Experimental rigor can be applied far more effectively by experimenters who work with biological or physical specimens, and who can more easily control the variables to analyze their experimental results.

Finally, we must remember that even a slight improvement in a condition may be significant to the individuals with that condition even though the treatment may not be statistically significant as far as a controlled experiment is concerned.

Thus far, we have referred frequently to the word *control,* which can be defined as a manipulation or alteration of the experimental conditions in order to limit sources of error.

As described in Chapter 4, the idea of experimental research is to determine if condition X (the cause) will result in response Y (the effect). Condition X is termed the *independent variable,* and response Y is the *dependent variable.*

The nature of control is to restrict the effects of extraneous variables that could have an impact upon the variables under investigation and affect the outcome of the research.

Careful controls are also used to avoid side effects that could occur during the course of a potentially harmful experiment. Many useful drugs may be highly toxic or have unpleasant side effects if dosages are too large. For example, experiments with rats and mice by the Food and Drug Administration have caused great furor by identifying artificial sweeteners, such as cyclamates and saccharin, as potential carcinogens. These experiments were conducted in such a manner that the quantities of potentially harmful substances to be ingested by the experimental animals were carefully controlled. By varying the quantity levels of the substances, the experimenters could determine differential responses to the substances. Also, while not being able to cite a specific relationship, the Surgeon General's reports are able to state that the more one smokes, the greater the odds are of having various medical problems.

Probably the most important control the experimenter utilizes is that of random assignments of subjects to groups (also called randomization). Every subject has an equal chance of being assigned to any group as the investigator assigns subjects to a control or experimental group on a random basis. The purpose of random assignment is to avoid any systematic bias in the groups concerning the variables being studied.

Experimental Research Designs

There are a number of ways to design experimental research. Each design is characterized by manipulation of the independent variable by the experimenter, and by some form of control. The designs range from quite simple to extremely complex. You will find it helpful to refer to the comparisons of experimental designs (Table 9-1) as each design is discussed.

One Group Pretest–Posttest Design

The simplest type of experimental design is the One Group Pretest–Posttest design. Although this is not a truly experimental research design because it leaves many things to chance, it is often the only available way to attempt to determine the effectiveness of a treatment. Essentially, this design measures what has happened to the experimental group based on the way it was prior to the beginning of the experiment (pretest state), and the differences achieved at the end of the experiment (posttest state).

For example, such a design might be utilized to study a group of patients who suffer mild angina pain. The experimenter could measure cholesterol levels in the patients' blood, and then ask the patients to restrict their intake of cholesterol through changes in their diets. After a given period of time, the experimenter would determine whether or not the mild angina pain had been reduced and if blood cholesterol levels had dropped. If blood cholesterol levels had dropped and angina pain had been reduced, the experimenter might then conclude that lowering cholesterol levels in the blood reduces angina pain. Note that there is minimal control placed on other variables that might be affecting the evidence of angina in the study subjects. Changes in stress patterns, weight, exercise patterns, or any one of many other factors might have contributed to the change.

Pretest–Posttest Control Group

A second and far more sophisticated technique of experimentation is the use of a control group to determine if the treatment appears to make a difference. Utilizing the previous cholesterol example, a number of subjects with mild angina pain would be randomly assigned to two groups: an *experimental group* and a *control group*. The experimental group subjects would then alter their diets, while the control group subjects would change nothing. At the end of the experiment, the researcher would then determine whether or not there was a significant difference in the cholesterol levels of both groups. If this difference was significant, and if there was a significant difference in the incidence of mild angina pain in the subjects in the experimental group but not in the control group, the experimenter could then conclude that reduction of blood cholesterol did have an effect on the occurrence of angina.

Please note that there has been no attempt to match or otherwise compare the members of either group. The only common element of control the control group shares with the experimental group is mild angina pain. Note also the term *mild.* Pain perception varies greatly from individual to individual, and response to pain varies between cultures as well as between the sexes in different cultures. All of these factors were not taken into consideration in the previous example, only the common diagnosis of mild angina pain.

Matching Samples

Far more valuable, in terms of rigor, would be the design by the researcher that attempts to match or to pair the control and the experimental group. In the cholesterol study, the experimenter might utilize simple matching procedures such as height, weight, sex, age, smoking and nonsmoking, or such sophisticated measurements as psychological stress tests, projective techniques, or any one of literally dozens of methods in order to control for extraneous variables.

A major problem with this type of experimental design is that, unless the subject pool is infinitely large, the experimenter reduces the available sample with each matching or pairing situation. Males can only be matched with males. Age further reduces the sample size; it is entirely possible to reduce the sample down to two very well matched individuals. The problem then becomes one of a large enough sample size to be generalizable to the target population.

Solomon Four Group Design

A frequently utilized and highly valid experimental procedure is the *Solomon Four Group Design.* An experimenter using this methodology randomly divides the sample into four separate groups. Effectively, there are two experimental groups and two control groups.

The first experimental group receives the same procedures as in the pretest–posttest procedure. Subjects are randomly selected, pretested, given the appropriate treatment, and then given the posttest.

The first of the control groups is given the pretest, no treatment and the posttest. Up to this point, the Solomon design is precisely the same as the pretest–posttest control group design. However, group three is also defined as an experimental group. In our cholesterol example, it would consist of subjects diagnosed as having mild angina. They would not be given the pretest; that is, their cholesterol level would not be measured at all. However, they would receive the treatment; that is, their intake of cholesterol would be reduced and they would be given the appropriate blood tests at the end of the experimental period.

Subjects in the fourth group in the Solomon design would have nothing done until the posttest. They would not be pretested for cholesterol levels at the experiment's beginning and they would not receive any treatment. Only at the end of the experiment would their blood cholesterol level be measured (posttested), and then compared to the incidence of anginal pain in the other groups.

Since two of the groups have received the experimental treatment, (groups 1 and 3), any differences noted by the experimenter can be more confidently ascribed to the treatment if both experimental groups show similar results at the end of the treatment and there is a significant difference between the experimental and control groups. Similarly, a lack of significant difference between the four groups enables the investigator to accept the null hypothesis.

Two Group Random Sample

The experimenter may choose to use only the last two groups of the Solomon design. That is, one group is given the treatment and then posttested with no pretesting, and the control group is given only the posttest. The theory of this methodology is that the experimenter, adhering rigorously to the random assignment of subjects to the groups, can say that the two groups were essentially the same because random assignment should avoid any systematic bias in the two groups.

This type of design simplifies the experimenter's tasks

and eliminates the effect of a pretest on the subjects. In effect, it maintains the subjects' naivete. It is also noteworthy that there are some things that cannot be pretested or accurately predicted. Patients who are already suffering from mild angina pains may or may not be suffering from elevated cholesterol levels. The angina pain already exists. If treatment or lack of treatment (cholesterol in the diet) is a factor, there should be a difference between the two groups at the end of the treatment.

Nonrandomized Control Group Design

Occasionally, circumstances may preclude random assignment of subjects to groups at the beginning of an experiment. For example, the experimenter may wish to compare a sample of individuals from a local Veteran's Administration hospital, who are complaining of angina pain, with a sample of individuals from a privately funded hospital, who are also complaining of angina pain. One of the hospitals may insist on a standardized routine of treatment for angina patients while the other hospital may be available for the experimental treatment.

In this case, the subjects in both samples are given the pretest and one group is given the experimental treatment, but the researcher is not able to control various interaction effects at the beginning of the experiment. In this instance where it is not possible to develop controls by assigning subjects randomly to control and experimental groups, alternative methods of statistical analysis are required. The method commonly utilized is the analysis of covariance. This statistical technique allows the experimenter to control for varying potential interaction effects after the experiment has been performed. Because this technique is quite involved, we strongly recommend that beginning researchers pursuing this type of design be very cautious and seek help from their instructor, or other qualified individual, prior to the data analysis.

Counter Balanced Design

A more effective design, or at least one that attempts to re-move some of the previously described problems, is the *Counter Balanced* design. This design can be used when more than one treatment method is attempted. Each set of subjects is given the treatment at the same point in time during the course of the experiment. This means that sets of subjects become both experimental and control for them-selves and for another group. Because of the nonrandom nature of group assignments, the experimenter cannot con-trol differences. However, the testing does allow for greater flexibility in the interpretation of results: differences are noted between groups and within groups. Utilizing the sta-tistical test of analysis of variance, the experimenter may be able to determine that the effects were caused by the treat-ment.

For example, a group of psychiatric patients might be subjected to a computerized program designed to interact with individuals and give the illusion of eliciting feelings. (Such a program exists as a novelty on many college com-puses and is often called "Doctor".) The subjects would then be given a subjective test after such interaction and their responses scored. At an alternate time, standard psychothera-peutic techniques would be utilized and the same projective tests would be given. After a number of alternating treat-ments, types of responses to the projective tests could be measured and the differences, if any, between the two treat-ments could be noted.

A number of variations to this design should be noted. Two or more variables could be introduced, such as another type of treatment in addition to computer and psychother-apy. Perhaps a questionnaire could be introduced utilizing a format such as "I feel ———————————." The sub-ject chooses from a list of adjectives provided and the subject is then asked to tell why he or she feels this way. Or, a ques-tion such as "How do you feel about ———————?" could be asked. Responses to projective techniques could again be used to determine differences between the treatments.

Time Series Design

Most experimental studies fall into two categories: the one shot study and those which continue over a longer period of time (longitudinal). As an experimenter you may want to measure the effects of a treatment over a long period of time. You would thus continue to administer the treatment and measure the effects a number of times during the course of the experiment.

In our cholesterol example, instead of testing patients with mild angina pain only once (at the end of the diet restriction), the design would call for multiple testing at stated intervals. Such a design would be far more desirable than the single pretest–posttest design which was initially described. Chemical or behavioral changes in a human being can be very subtle to measure. Responses can vary daily and some intervening, but unrecognized, variables may lead to an incorrect conclusion. Testing over a long period of time helps to reduce such pitfalls and enhances the experiment. With a time series experiment, however, variables may occur during and after treatment that may be unnoticed by the experimenter and can lead to a false or improper conclusion.

Control Group Time Series Design

In order to diminish the problems inherent in a time series design, experimenters can utilize a *Control Group Time Series Design*. This design requires that a control group be tested simultaneously with the experimental group without being given the treatment. In our cholesterol example, two groups of randomly selected angina patients would receive a sequential series of blood tests over a period of time. The experimenter would then determine if blood cholesterol had diminished significantly between the experimental treatment group and the control group, as well as the frequency and intensity of angina pain. This technique, obviously, provides far greater control than a single time series design and is preferable to the single time series design.

Factorial Designs

In experimental designs such as we have been discussing, the experimenter identifies one independent variable and one dependent variable. Through the use of various forms of control, the effect of the independent variable on the dependent variable is then measured. However, there may be a time when we find there are two or more variables that have occurred simultaneously and, through interaction, may cause the dependent variable to appear in the way it did.

Using our cholesterol example, suppose the subjects were overweight when placed on the low cholesterol diet. In some cases weight might be maintained because, while saturated fat intake is reduced, there is a plethora of nonsaturated fats which could be substituted for the saturated fat.

However, the experimenter might want to reduce both the weight and the intake of saturated fats of the subjects simultaneously. At the end of the experiment, it might be found that angina pain had been reduced in intensity and frequency. It would then become very difficult to ascribe the causal effects to the two independent variables. Experimenters can more easily control experiments where there is one and only one independent variable introduced, such as in the case of a cholesterol intake reduction alone or a weight loss diet alone. Often the interaction of two or more variables produces more significant results than a single variable does. The experimenter, then, must use what is called a *Factorial Design*. In this type of design, subjects are divided into all possible combinations to determine the effect of the independent variables alone and the effect of the interaction of the independent variables.

Such factorial designs can grow to enormous complexity very quickly, but such is the work of researchers. Human beings are enormously complex and even the simplest, most tightly designed and tightly controlled experiment has results that are probably influenced by interaction effects. Factorial designs attempt to get at these interactive effects and determine their impact on the experiment.

Ex Post Facto Designs–Correlations

In ex post facto research, changes in the independent variable have already occurred prior to the research. Ex post facto designs are really correlational designs that allow the researcher to infer relationships among variables, rather than draw cause and effect conclusions. This can lead to spurious (incorrect) conclusions. Researchers who conclude that a high positive or a high negative correlation is necessarily a cause and effect relationship have failed to see the whole picture. There is a tendency to oversimplify in drawing conclusions. It has been said that there are two solutions to every problem: one short, simple, and wrong, and the other extremely complicated. Indeed, there has been a problem regarding the reports of several regulatory agencies of the Federal government, such as the Food and Drug Administration and the Surgeon General's office, both of which have reported a great deal of correlational research. Because of the potential ambiguity in interpretation, industries such as the tobacco industry or the artificial sweetener industry have often attempted—and sometimes succeeded—in responding to these reports with other correlational studies of their own showing lower relationships or no causality at all. This has led to much confusion on the consumer's part because the question of whom to believe looms large when dealing with such complex marketplace issues.

Considerations in Experimental Research Design

In all true experimental studies, the researcher must keep several concerns as high priority items when designing research.

Table 9–1 Comparison of Experimental Designs

Design	Number of Groups	Pretest		Treatment		Posttest		Level of Value (Weak/Strong)
One Group pretest/Posttest	One		Yes		Yes		Yes	Weak
Pretest/Posttest Control Group	Two	X	Yes	X	Yes	X	Yes	Weak
		C	Yes	C	No	C	Yes	
Matching Samples	Two	X	Yes	X	Yes	X	Yes	Weak
		C	No	C	No	C	Yes	
Solomon Four Group Design	Four	X	Yes	X	Yes	X	Yes	Strong
		C	Yes	C	Yes	C	Yes	
		X	No	X	No	C	Yes	
		C	No	C	No			
Two Group Random Sample	Two	X	No	X	Yes	X	Yes	Strong
		C	No	C	No	C	Yes	
Non randomized Control Group	Two	X	Yes	X	Yes	X	Yes	Control through analysis of covariance can be strong
		C	Yes	C	No	C	Yes	

Counter Balanced	Varies—Xs & Ys reverse roles in study	X Yes C Yes X Yes C Yes	X Yes C No	X Yes C Yes	Strong
Time Series	One	Yes	Yes over time repeated measures	Yes over time repeated measures	Strong
Control Group Time Series	Two	X Yes C Yes	X Yes over time C No over time	X Yes over time C Yes over time	Strong
Factorial	Varies	X Yes C Varies	X Yes C Varies	X Yes C Yes	Strong but can be very complex

Generalizability

Insofar as possible, the researcher should design the experiment so that its findings will be generalizable to the larger target population when sampling techniques are used. Sometimes research studies do not allow for generalization because of sample size, method of selection, or various other reasons. In addition, experiments conducted in artificial or restricted laboratory situations often preclude generalization.

Subject Sensitization

Subjects can become sensitized or knowledgeable about the procedures used. This is especially true where some kind of psychological rather than physiological response is measured. By its very nature, a pretest gives information about what it is that the experimenter wants to discover. Even if questions are masked, subjects will know something about the research. Even physiological measurements can be affected. With the increase of knowledge of biofeedback we can see that subjects may control, voluntarily or involuntarily, many of their physiological responses.

Historical Factors

Historical factors may also come into play. If an experiment is carried out over a period of time, events extraneous to the experiment such as maturation or increased knowledge may cause changes. These events become intervening variables and must be accounted for.

Fatigue

Both the subjects and the researchers can become fatigued, bored, or inattentive during the course of a research project. This means treatment, or response measurement, may not be consistent during the course of an experiment. There comes a time in almost any experiment or research project when both subjects and researchers have the feeling of "let's get this thing over with and get out of here." This natural fatigue has to be guarded against in order to insure correct and consistent measurement.

Attrition

In research conducted over a period of time, there may be attrition or a loss of subjects. Subjects move, become ill, withdraw because they are tired of the research or are lost to the experiment for any number of reasons. This means that an experimenter who starts with too small a sample or samples at the beginning of the experiment may obtain insufficient data for valid analysis.

Hawthorne Effect

There have been many studies of the *Hawthorne Effect* over the years. The Hawthorne studies were a series of classic experimental studies conducted in the late 1920s and early 1930s at the Hawthorne Plant of the Western Electric Company in Chicago. The *Hawthorne Effect* is the term used to describe the psychological reactions to the presence of the investigator or to special treatment during the study which tends to alter the responses of the subjects. Subjects may change their behavior and try to please the experimenter. Frequently, the subject will attempt to give the response he or she believes will please the experimenter. Again, we caution you that experimenters can unconsciously bias subjects merely by the tone of their voices or their facial expressions.

Experimenter Bias

Sometimes experimenter expectations interfere with the gathering of accurate results. Many experimenters have a vested interest in their experiments, and the failure to disprove the null hypothesis may be a terrible blow to one's ego. A true researcher remains objective and attempts to control as many variables as possible.

Summary

In summary, we have discussed a number of the most commonly used research designs including: the one group pretest–posttest design; the pretest–posttest control group design; matching sample design; Solomon Four Group Design; Two Group Random Sample design; Nonrandom control group design; counter balanced design; time series design; control group time series design and factorial designs. We also discussed ex post facto designs–correlations. Beginning researchers should be aware that there are other less common designs which may be found in the literature.

In order to apply the principles presented, you should complete the Application Activities listed below.

Application Activities

1. Reread the experimental research report in Appendix A. Note how the experimenters defined the experimental controls, population and sample size.
2. Reread the experimental research proposal in Appendix D and the completed research report in Appendix E.
3. Find two published experimental research reports; determine which type of experimental design was utilized.

Bibliography and Suggested Readings

Campbell, Donald T., and Stanley, Julian. *Experimental and Quasi Experimental Designs for Research*. Chicago: Rand McNally, 1963.

Forcese, Dennis P.; Richer, Stephen. *Social Research Methods*. Englewood Cliffs, N.J.: Prentice-Hall, 1973.

Kerlinger, Fred H. *Foundations of Behavioral Research*, 2nd ed. New York: Holt, Rinehart and Winston, 1973.

Leedy, Paul D. *Practical Research: Planning and Design*. New York: Macmillan, 1974.

Selltiz, Claire; Wrightsman, Lawrence; Cook, Stephen. *Research Methods in Social Relations,* 3rd ed. New York: Holt, Rinehart and Winston, 1976.

Solomon, Richard C. "An Extension of Control Group Design," *Psychological Bulletin* 46 (1949):137–150.

Van Dalen, Deobold B. *Understanding Educational Research,* 3rd ed. New York: McGraw-Hill, 1973.

Wiseman, Jacqueline P.; Aron, Marcia S. *Field Projects for Sociology Students.* Cambridge, Mass.: Schenkman Publishing, 1970.

Appendix A

REPRINT OF A PUBLISHED
NURSING RESEARCH STUDY

Topical Application of Insulin in Decubitus Ulcers

Rose Marie Gerber • Suzanne Rowe Van Ort

When a pilot study provided evidence that insulin may increase the rate of healing of decubitus ulcers, this study attempted to answer the question: Is topical insulin therapy an effective treatment regimen for decubitus ulcers? The experimental study utilized a two-group, before–after design. Twenty-nine geriatric subjects were randomly assigned to either the experimental or the control group. The single independent variable was the topical application of ten units of regular insulin (U.S.P.) twice daily. The dependent variable was the surface area of the decubitus ulcer measured in square millimeters. Rate of healing was defined as decrease in surface area over time. Data were also gathered on extraneous variables believed to influence the healing process. The F test was used to test the research hypothesis that experimental subjects would have an increased rate of healing. When comparison of group means on day seven and day 15 revealed no significant differences, the research hypothesis was rejected. Pearson product moment correlation procedures were utilized to determine if there were differences between extraneous variables and the rate of healing. Females healed significantly ($p < .05$) more slowly than males. Also, there was a direct correlation between the number of days of treatment and the rate of healing.

THE purpose of this study was to evaluate further topical insulin therapy as a treatment regimen for decubitus ulcers. A pilot study by Van Ort and Gerber (1976) provided evidence that insulin may increase the rate of healing of decubitus ulcers.

Rationale. Wound healing depends on the provision or restoration of local circulation and cellular reproduction or tissue repair. The formation and deposition of collagen, an integral part of cellular reproduction and connective tissue formation, involves protein as building blocks. Therefore, adequate protein synthesis is a primary requisite to satisfactory wound healing and tissue repair.

The protein molecule is chemically synthesized from amino acids, and it is believed that insulin may enhance amino acid transport into the cells (Guyton, 1976). It would seem, then, that insulin could influence the rate of wound healing.

The exact biochemical or pharmacologic mechanisms of topical insulin therapy, i.e., whether exogenous or endogenous mechanisms are involved, remains unclear. Guyton stated that a lack of insulin reduces protein synthesis to

almost zero. Other researchers reported the beneficial effects of insulin in wound healing (Grewal et al., 1972; Sedlarik, 1969; Stirewalt et al., 1967; and Udupa and Chansouria, 1971). Although the healing process in decubitus ulcers may be protracted or imperfect, the sequence of events involves the same physiologic processes of tissue repair. And regardless of the exact biochemical mechanism involved, insulin could be expected to have a positive effect on the healing process of decubitus ulcers.

Review of the Literature. The literature supports the study of topical insulin therapy from physiologic and thera-

peutic standpoints. Earlier works include histologic studies in animals as well as the study of human subjects.

Sedlarik (1969) used watering therapy in a treatment regimen for promoting healing of ulcerated wounds. He used a drip method to apply, in sequence, a hypertonic solution, an insulin solution, and a hypotonic solution. Following treatment with the prescribed therapy, he reported evidence of successful healing in all 28 human subjects in the study.

Of particular significance to the present study was a report by Paul (1966) of a case study in which topical insulin was used effectively to treat a chronic and infected skin ulcer in a 56-year-old diabetic woman. A piece of gauze was soaked with 20 units (I.U.) of soluble insulin, placed over the wound, and covered by a bandage. This local application was repeated twice daily. No antibiotics were given during this treatment with insulin. With time the wound healed completely. Hughey (1974) found that topical insulin had a positive

ROSE MARIE GERBER (Massilon City Hospital School of Nursing, Massillon; M.S., Ohio State University, Columbus, Ohio) is associate professor, College of Nursing, University of Arizona, Tucson.

SUZANNE ROWE VAN ORT (University of Arizona School of Nursing, Tucson; Ph.D., University of Arizona, Tucson) is dean, School of Nursing, University of Wisconsin—Eau Claire.

effect on the healing of chronic skin ulcerations in diabetics.

Since the major problem of decubitus ulcers involves the healing process, insulin may be of value. The healing process in decubitus ulcers involves the same physiologic process as in secondary union. Therefore, it seems logical to assume that if insulin enhances wound healing in one situation, it would also be beneficial in others.

Hypothesis. The research hypothesis tested was that there would be a significant increase in the rate of healing of the decubitus ulcers in subjects who received 10 units (I.U.) of regular insulin (U.S.P.) topically twice daily.

Method. *Subjects.* The target population was composed of local nursing home residents. Although it was proposed to include 40 subjects, only 31 were available for study. Criteria for selection of subjects included: a break in skin continuity as evidenced by epidermal or dermal injury involving erythe-

ma, pallor, cyanosis, and superficial erosion; size of the ulcer at the time the subject was admitted to the study measured between 1.0 and 7.0 cm; skin breakdown had been in evidence three days or less prior to the time the subject was admitted to the study.

Of the 31 subjects, two were dropped because their ulcer measurements were so much larger than the other 29 that they spuriously skewed the data. Sixteen of the remaining 29 subjects were in the experimental group; 13, in the control group.

Research Design. The study followed an experimental model and utilized a two-group, before–after design. Subjects were randomly assigned to experimental and control groups. Subjects in both groups were pretested by measurement of the ulcer surface area and retested every day for 15 days.

All subjects received routine supportive nursing care. This care included position changes, hygienic measures, fluid and protein intake, and local mas-

sage. Only subjects in the experimental group received insulin therapy. Subjects in the control group were treated with any of a variety of specific decubitus ulcer therapies other than insulin.

Variables. The single independent variable consisted of dropping ten units (I.U.) of U-40 regular insulin (U.S.P.) from a syringe. The ulcer was then allowed to dry. No dressing was applied. The dependent variable was the rate of healing of the decubitus ulcer as evidenced by a change in the size (mm^2) of the ulcer surface area.

Extraneous variables which were assessed prior to the subject's participation in the study included: fasting blood glucose, hemoglobin, nutrition (estimated fluid and protein intake per day), mobility/activity, continency, medical diagnosis, medications, body weight (underweight, normal, or overweight), age, sex, number and location(s) of decubitus ulcers.

Instrumentation. Based on recommendations of the pilot study (Van Ort and Gerber, 1976), the method for measuring the decutitus ulcer was changed in order to enhance precision.

The surface area of the decubitus ulcer was measured in square millimeters. A piece of waxed paper was placed over the decubitus ulcer and an outline of the ulcer was traced on the waxed paper. The completed tracing was then transferred to graph paper calibrated in square millimeters for calculation of surface area.

Data Collection. All topical insulin therapy and all data collection were done by trained research assistants who were graduate nursing students. All other care was provided by the nursing staff. Initially, the investigator identified potential subjects by progressing from lower numbered rooms in the nursing home to higher numbered rooms. When subjects met the criteria, the investigator talked with the subject, explained the study, and obtained written consent. The subject's physician was consulted and the necessary medical orders obtained. Subjects were then continuously assigned according to a table of random numbers to experimental or control group.

The subject's hemoglobin was drawn and measured by a clinical laboratory. The subject's fasting blood glucose was measured in the nursing home utilizing an Ames' Eyetone Reflectance Colorimeter.[1] The blood glucose procedure required a single drop of blood on a Dextrostix® reagent.

For subjects in the experimental group, the following activities occurred sequentially: On the first day, the preprocedural assessment was done, the decubitus ulcer was measured, and a fasting blood glucose level obtained. The insulin therapy was then initiated. Because the possible absorption of insulin through the ulcer was not well documented in the literature, the University Human Subjects committee requested that all insulin treatments be done at mealtime. Therefore, all insulin therapy

[1] Manufactured by the Ames Company, Elkhart, Indiana.

was applied immediately before breakfast and before the evening meal. Two hours after the insulin treatment, another blood glucose was obtained to determine if the insulin had caused hypoglycemia.

On the second through fifth days, the decubitus ulcer was measured once daily and the insulin applied twice daily. Use of a five-day therapy protocol was based on earlier clinical experience.

From the sixth through the 14th days, the decubitus ulcer was measured and observed once daily. In the event that ulcer surface area increased by 50 mm or more during any 24-hour period, the insulin regimen was reapplied for another five days. On the 15th day the final decubitus ulcer measurement was taken.

For subjects in the control group, the first day's activities were the same as for subjects in the experimental group except that they received any specific decubitus ulcer treatment other than insulin therapy; choice of therapy was determined by the control subject's physician or by nursing home standing orders. The two-hour postprandial blood sugars were omitted for control subjects.

On the second through the 15th days, the decubitus was measured daily and nursing home personnel continued to treat the ulcer.

Informed Consent. The human rights aspect of this study was addressed in the following manner: 1) The investigator explained the purpose of the research and what was required of each participant; 2) subjects were given the right to refuse to participate in the research; 3) subjects were informed that the results of this research would be published but that their identity would remain anonymous; 4) subjects were informed that they could withdraw from the research at any time without prejudice; 5) subjects were advised of the costs, benefits, demands, and risks of the study; and 6) the investigator obtained the written consent of each subject.

Data Analysis. Both descriptive and inferential statistics were utilized to examine the data. The criterion for significance of the data consisted of the *F*-ratio to measure the differences between group means. Significance was set at $p<.05$. A one-way analysis of variance was performed to determine relationships between dependent and independent variables. A Pearson product moment correlation coefficient was computed to determine the relationship between the extraneous variables and the dependent variable. Finally, a multiple regression analysis was performed to delineate further the relationship between the extraneous variables and the dependent variables.

Results. *Description of the Population.* Twenty-one subjects were female. With one exception, all subjects were confined to either bed or chair. Twenty-three subjects were incontinent. Four subjects were diagnosed diabetics. All subjects experienced either constant or intermittent pressure on the site of the ulcer. A frequency distribution for extraneous variables scored on nominal scales is presented in Table 1. Central tendency and variability of selected extraneous variables are presented in Table 2.

The two groups of subjects were similar in relation to all extraneous variables except age. One-way analysis of variance by group revealed that the experimental group was significantly ($p<.05$) older. Pearson product moment correlation coefficients for extraneous variables also revealed a statistically significant ($p<.02$) age difference; subjects in the control group were younger (Table 3). Though not statistically different, control group subjects tended to be better nourished, to have higher hemoglobins, and to be more mobile. These factors may have been clinically significant.

Observation of Blood Glucose. Because some concern was related to the unknown absorption of insulin from the ulcer site, fasting blood glucose levels size of the ulcer over time. Table 5, the source table for one-way analyses of variance, shows no significant difference for group means of rate of healing on day seven and day 15. Because the ulcers on 19 of the 29 subjects completely healed to zero measurements within the 15-day study period, number of days to first zero was also used as an indicator of rate of healing. Again, there were no significant differences.

Extraneous Variables. Pearson product moment correlations were used to determine relationships between the extraneous variables and the rate of healing (see Table 6). Of extraneous variables studied, only sex was a significant factor in relation to rate of healing. Females healed significantly more slowly than males. Also, number of days of treatment varied as an artifact of the research design. A direct correlation between rate of healing and number of days of treatment was observed.

Pearson product moment correlations

Table 1. Frequency Distribution of Selected Extraneous Variables by Group and Total

EXTRANEOUS VARIABLES	GROUP		TOTAL (N=29)
	EXPERIMENTAL (N=16)	CONTROL (N=13)	
Body build			
Underweight	11	5	16
Normal	3	5	8
Overweight	2	3	5
Fluid intake[1]			
Less than 1000 ml.	8	4	12
1000-2000 ml.	7	6	13
2000-3000 ml.	1	3	4
More than 3000 ml.	0	0	0
Protein intake[1]			
Less than 30 Gm.	5	1	6
30-50 Gm.	6	5	11
More than 50 Gm.	5	7	12
Location of ulcer			
Sacrum	8	5	13
Buttocks	4	6	10
Trochanter	2	1	3
Heel	0	1	1
Shoulder	1	0	1
Thigh	1	0	1

[1] Approximate daily intake

were determined on all experimental patients prior to the first insulin treatment, which occurred at the time of breakfast, and then repeated two hours after the insulin treatment. Data are summarized in Table 4. If insulin was absorbed from the site of the ulcer, effects were canceled by the ingestion of breakfast.

Rate of Healing. The rate of healing was defined as the decrease in the mm²

Table 2. Central Tendency and Variability of Selected Extraneous Variables by Group and Total (N=29)

Extraneous Variables	Central Tendency			Variability	
	$\bar{X}$	Median	Mode	Range	S. D.
Age, in years					
Total (N=29)	81.172	81.000	76,82	68-96	6.342
Experimental (N=16)	83.438	83.500	—	73-96	6.373
Control (N=13)	78.385	78.000	76	68-86	4.755
Fasting blood glucose (mg.%)					
Total	77.897	70.250	65,85	45-190	29.358
Experimental	72.438	65.000	—	45-135	—
Control	84.615	75.000	65	55-190	—
Hemoglobin (Gm.%)					
Total	12.955	13.167	13.2	8.8-16.2	1.555
Experimental	12.588	12.850	13.2	8.8-16.2	1.810
Control	13.408	13.400	—	12.3-14.9	0.8939
Number of ulcers present					
Total	1.966	1.467	1	1-4	1.180
Experimental	2.125	1.740	1	1-4	—
Control	1.769	1.000	1	1-4	—

Table 3. Pearson Product Moment Correlation Coefficients of Extraneous Variables for Control Group with Experimental Group (N=29)

Extraneous Variables	Pearson r	Signif- icance
Age	-.4033	.015
Sex	-.0642	.370
Body build	.2668	.081
Fasting blood glucose	.2099	.137
Hemoglobin	.2670	.081
Daily fluid intake	.2600	.087
Daily protein intake	.3019	.056
Number of ulcers present	-.1526	.215
Mobility	.2956	.060
Incontinence	.2243	.121
Diagnosed diabetes	-.0416	.415

between extraneous variables and the number of days to first zero by group (Table 7) revealed in the experimental group a significant correlation between subject's age and number of days to first zero. As age increased, so did number of days for healing. In the control group there was a significant correlation between sex and number of days to first zero. Women healed more slowly.

There were also significant correlations between hemoglobin and rate of healing in both groups. In the experimental group there was a negative correlation; that is, as hemoglobin decreased, number of days to first zero increased. In the control group there was a positive correlation; as hemoglobin increased, number of days to first zero increased. There were also significant correlations be-

tween number of days of treatment and number of days to first zero in both groups.

The multiple regression analysis supported other statistical procedures and provided no additional information.

Discussion. When the F-test was used to test the research hypothesis that the experimental subjects would have an increased rate of healing, comparisons on days seven and 15 revealed differences in the direction sought, but the

Table 4. Comparison of Fasting and Posttreatment Blood Glucose Levels for Experimental Subjects (N=16)

Times of Testing	Blood Glucose Levels (in mg. %)			
	$\bar{X}$	Median	Range	S. D.
Fasting	72.438	65.500	45-135	23.446
Two-hour posttreatment	115.313	97.500	70-250	48.870

Table 5. Analysis of Variance Source Tables for Rate of Healing Day 7 and Day 15 between Groups

Source	df	S.S.	M.S.	F-Ratio	F-Probability
Day seven					
Between groups	1	3786.1597	3786.1597	2.132	.156
Within groups	27	47958.1192	1776.2266		
Total	28	51744.2789			
Day 15					
Between groups	1	1569.2217	1569.2217	.667	.421
Within groups	27	63564.9145	2354.2561		
Total	28	65134.1362	2354.2561		

differences were not significant. The research hypothesis was rejected. Because directionality was evident, an increased number of subjects may have more accurately reflected true differences.

There were consistent and significant positive correlations between number of days of treatment and rate of healing.

This finding was of particular interest in relation to the insulin therapy protocol which provided for only five days of therapy, unless the ulcer surface area increased. It appears that insulin therapy should be continued until healing has occurred. This study showed that topical insulin can be safely applied at mealtime.

Why did elderly women who were treated with the topical insulin therapy heal significantly more slowly than men? Could there be hormonal-insulin interactions in postmenopausal females? Would younger females respond the same way? These questions remain unanswered.

The question regarding the effectiveness of topical insulin therapy as a treatment regimen for decubitus ulcers remains unclear. The observed clinical effectiveness of insulin therapy was not supported by this study.

Recommendations for Further Study. Because of clinical experiences in the use of topical insulin in the treatment of decubitus ulcers and because of encouraging results with a relatively small number of subjects, study of the problem should be continued.

Based on the findings of this study, the following recommendations are suggested for consideration in future work: Control for the sex factor should be implemented. Control for age-related factors which may influence the rate of healing is necessary. Younger subjects who are physiologically different from subjects in this study should be tested. Additional study is needed to document effective and safe dosages of topical insulin. It appears that ten units of insulin is a minimal dose and questions can still be raised regarding absorption of insulin through the ulcerated tissue. Biochemical research of cellular reactions to topical insulin therapy is imperative. In the future topical insulin therapy should continue until the ulcer is healed. Improved instrumentation to measure healing of ulcers (granulation) is also needed. The lesion-size measure used in the pilot study lacked precision; in larger ulcers the number of mm² became magnified and were difficult to manage statistically. Perhaps a classification system is needed to show overall changes over time.

Also, in clinical practice, decubitus ulcers were cleansed with hydrogen peroxide before the insulin was applied. This aspect of the treatment was discon-

Table 6. Pearson Product Moment Correlations of Selected Extraneous Variables with Indexes of Healing Rate (N=29)

EXTRANEOUS VARIABLES	SIZE OF ULCER			HEALING RATE	
	DAY 1	DAY 7	DAY 15	DAY 7	DAY 15
Age	-.0071 (.485)	-.0237 (.451)	-.0241 (.451)	-.0196 (.460)	-.0222 (.454)
Sex	-.1047 (.294)	-.5254 (.002)	-.5266 (.002)	-.4127 (.013)	-.4695 (.005)
Fasting blood glucose	.0438 (.411)	.0120 (.475)	-.1529 (.214)	.0264 (.446)	-.1122 (.281)
Hemoglobin	-.0557 (.387)	-.1032 (.297)	-.0279 (.443)	-.0955 (.311)	-.0412 (.416)
Number of days of treatment	.3479 (.032)	.6118 (.001)	.4097 (.014)	.5733 (.001)	.4517 (.007)

Table 7. Pearson Product Moment Correlation Coefficients by Group for Extraneous Variables with Number of Days to First Zero

EXTRANEOUS VARIABLES	EXPERIMENTAL GROUP (N=16)		CONTROL GROUP (N=13)	
	r	SIGNIFICANCE	r	SIGNIFICANCE
Age	.4994	.024	-.0085	.489
Sex	.1444	.297	-.4770	.050
Body build	-.1744	.259	-.3631	.111
Blood glucose	-.0141	.479	.0750	.404
Hemoglobin	-.5187	.020	.5216	.034
Fluid intake	.2603	.165	.2303	.255
Protein intake	.2712	.310	-.0858	.390
Number of ulcers	.1341	.155	-.4016	.087
Mobility	.3287	.107	-.1398	.324
Incontinence	.1486	.291	.0103	.487
Diabetes mellitus	-.0946	.364	-.1771	.281
Number of days of treatment	.4187	.053	.6452	.009

tinued for research purposes. However, in retrospect it appears that the hydrogen peroxide may have provided some useful cleansing and debridement. Future study should include topical application of hydrogen peroxide as a part of the topical insulin therapy.

A survey should determine the extent of clinical use of topical insulin therapy. It would be helpful to know: 1) the geographic use of topical insulin therapy, 2) treatment protocols, 3) kinds of clinical problems treated with topical insulin, and 4) an opinion or assessment of the effectiveness of the therapy. ∦

References

GREWAL, R. S., AND OTHERS. Wound healing in relation to insulin. *Int Surg* 57:229-232, Mar. 1972.

GUYTON, A. C. *Textbook of Medical Physiology.* 5th ed. Philadelphia, W. B. Saunders Co., 1976.

HUGHEY, J. R. *A Comparison of the Treatment of the Diabetic with Topical Insulin and the Light Cradle.* Tucson, Department of Pharmacology, College of Medicine, University of Arizona, 1974. (Unpublished masters thesis)

PAUL, T. N. Treatment by local application of insulin of an infected wound in a diabetic. *Lancet* 2:574-576, Sept. 10, 1966.

SEDLARIK, K. (Local wound treatment in diabetes mellitus.) (German) *Zentralbl Chir* 94:209-217, Feb. 15, 1969.

STIREWALT, W. S., AND OTHERS. Relation of RNA and protein synthesis to the sedimentation of muscle ribosomes: Effect of diabetes and insulin. *Proc Natl Acad Sci USA* 57:1885-1892, June 1967.

UDUPA, K. N., AND CHANSOURIA, J. P. The role of protamine zinc insulin in accelerating wound healing in the rat. *Br J Surg* 58:673-675. Sept. 1971.

VAN ORT, S. R., AND GERBER, R. M. Topical application of insulin in the treatment of decubitus ulcers: A pilot study. *Nurs Res* 25:9-12, Jan.-Feb. 1976.

Appendix B

EXAMPLE OF A HISTORICAL RESEARCH PROPOSAL: "MARY BRECKINRIDGE, R.N.: A PROFILE"

By
Ironaca Morris
(Used with Permission)

Table of Contents

Introduction and Statement of the Problem

Historical research in nursing is an area that has developed slowly. Valuable information about nursing leaders has not been documented and may be lost to the profession and to posterity. People in society make events happen which promote change, and thus history is made. The nursing profession has a responsibility to single out those nurses who have contributed to the development and advancement of nursing in the areas of education, practice, and research. In planning for progress with a futuristic approach it is important to examine the contributions of past eras. A basic difference between the most primitive society and the industrial or technologically advanced societies is the sense of history and records that are available to the modern man. Growth occurs when the relevance of historic events is considered and facts examined in the light of present advances in knowledge.

Nursing is a major focus of contact between people and the health delivery services. Forces that affect people in society have an impact on health care and flexibility is required to cope with those changes. The need for studies in the history of nursing has been stated as a priority by the Commission on Nursing Research of the American Nurses' Association.[1] This historical research could serve as a guide-

---

1. American Nurses' Association, *Priorities for Research in Nursing,* Code No. D-51 3M. (Kansas City: The Association, May 1976).

post for others in identifying needed areas for future research.

Literature Review

The goal of providing quality health care to this nation is still a major problem because of inaccessibility, unavailability, and maldistribution of resources for health care. This dilemma, combined with the escalating costs of hospital care, poses a challenge for this decade. These factors existed in the Appalachian region of southeastern Kentucky, a vast forested area inhabited by some 10,000 people. There was no motor road within 60 miles in any direction and the only modes of travel were horseback and mule team. This describes the territory of the Frontier Nursing Service that Mrs. Mary Breckinridge surveyed in 1920 as she rode through the area to learn from the people what their greatest needs were and how they could be met. The social and economic conditions in this beautiful part of America were well below the poverty level. The maternal and infant mortality rates were high even for the county, while medical services were non-existent in the area. Mrs. Breckinridge was highly motivated and used her energies to find a solution for rendering health assistance. The solution she proposed was to use the nurse–midwife to deliver the needed care. Thus, the Frontier Nursing Service became the first organization in America to use nurses qualified as midwives. Her altruism and organizational abilities were prime factors in developing this model of health care delivery. It was patterned after the midwifery services used in the Scottish Highlands. Mrs. Breckinridge's work is well documented by the history and work of the Frontier Nursing Service.

The experiment in the Appalachians of Kentucky has received worldwide publicity because it succeeded in its goals. There is a need for further research into the health care delivery model as it relates to size, community participation, the low cost of home care, and the job satisfaction of the staff members. The leadership qualities of Mary Breckinridge and her acumen should be an inspiration to all nurses who aspire to become change agents.

Statement of the Purpose of the Study

The purpose of this study is to contribute to the history of nursing by portraying the personality and accomplishments of Mary Breckinridge, a nurse–midwife (1881–1965), and her contributions to nursing and to nurse–midwifery practice.

Definition of Terms

Nurse–midwifery practice is the independent management of care of essentially normal newborns and women, antepartally, intrapartally, postpartally and/or gynecologically. It occurs within a health care system that provides for medical consultation, collaborative management, or referral and is in accord with the *Functions, Standards, and Qualifications for Nurse–Midwifery Practice* as defined by the American College of Nurse–Midwives.[2]

Infant mortality rate is the number of children per 1,000 live births who die before their first birthday.

Maternity mortality rate refers to the number of mothers who die per 100,000 live births.

Methodology

The profile of Mrs. Breckinridge and her contribution to nursing will be organized to include the following data:

1. Personal data:
   To include date, place of birth, general family background, early influences, early education.
2. Personality and characteristics:
   a. Leadership qualities, b. personal attributes

---

2. American College of Nurse–Midwives, *What Is a Nurse–Midwife?* (Washington, D.C.: American College of Nurse–Midwives, 1978).

3. Professional education:
   a. Basic R.N., b. post-basic and certificate courses, c. degrees
4. Philosophy:
   a. Of life, b. of people, c. of nursing
5. Achievements:
   a. Personal, b. professional
6. Social relationships with:
   a. Friends, b. professional colleagues

This historical study will require the researcher to visit the Frontier Nursing Service in Kentucky to review their archives. Appointments for interviews and discussions will be scheduled in writing before departure. The focus will include local organizations, local and national newspaper copies, and the archivist. A prepared list of bibliographic references taken from the literature search will enable the researcher to focus on those areas of maximal import to the study.

The historical research design will be used, and the data will be subjected to intense and critical scrutiny. Sources used will include manuscripts, official records, laws, letters, minutes of meetings, eyewitness accounts, newspapers, stories, articles, diaries, biographies, as well as taped oral histories and films. Permission to use private documents and illustrations or photographs will need to be obtained.

Both primary and secondary data sources will be used. The major emphasis in this research will be the examination of information written by Mrs. Breckinridge, providing direct evidence of her specific experiences and reactions to the conditions existing at that time. Therefore, her autobiography, *Wide Neighborhoods,* and articles authored by her, will be used as the primary sources of data. Factual information, before it is used, must be corroborated by other primary sources. Data with only one corroborating primary source will be seen as a probability. Material is categorized as a possibility when events described are supported by sufficient evidence from secondary sources, but no corroborating primary source can be located.

Validation of unpublished letters and journals will be carried out by the researcher by subjecting data to the process of external criticism. This can be seen by the questions the researcher must answer: What is the origin of the manuscript? Where, when, why and by whom was it written? Is this document a fraud? Comparison of letters and signatures for handwriting is necessary, as well as letterheads and postmarks to prove possible, probable or factual authorship. Is it the original or a copy? Copies of documents will have to be compared to the original to avoid recurring copying errors. Is there uncertainty about the time of the documentation? Is it dated? Who is the author? Could it have been wirtten by Mrs. Breckinridge at this time?

When a document has been validated according to the described criteria, the next step is to examine the data for reliability, using the method of internal criticism. For this to be positive, it is necessary to understand the statements in the documents, avoiding personal biases and projected meanings. Colloquial terms will be used in some of these documents as the Kentucky area is rich in folk culture. These terms will require interpretation in the context of the customs and time in which the work was written. After positive criticism comes the next phase, negative criticism, when the researcher focuses attention on verifying the accuracy of the statements. Firsthand reports by eye or ear witnesses will be considered most reliable.

Secondary sources to be used involve materials obtained from others. Information is often contained in books and articles that were obtained by the author from a primary source, but in reporting it is subjected to her perceptions. Documentation of the personal characteristics of Mrs. Breckinridge will be done from the secondary sources, as others saw her. Thus, all information obtained for use in the historical research must pass the criteria of internal and external criticism for reliability and validity, respectively.

Limitations of the Study

Personal bias, projection of meanings, and wrong interpretation of facts can pose a real problem to the researcher.

In the collection and synthesis of the data, it is necessary to maintain an open mind combined with objectivity and a certain amount of skepticism to avoid being "carried away." The following example illustrates the problem. The dates for Mrs. Breckinridge's widowhood and births of her two children are not recorded in the literature reviewed, except in *Who Was Who in America*.[3] The impression could be formed that Mrs. Breckinridge was unmarried before entering hospital training. Further research and verification is indicated. Consideration should be given at this time to the fact that she spent much of her time outside of the mountains in the early years, developing a basis of financial support that survived the depression and enabled the service to carry on in the ensuing years.[4] This statement is fraught with possibilities, and valid, reliable documentation will support it if it is included in the research report. In view of the social background and the role and status of women at that time, it may be necessary to show that she was not enjoying the bright lights of society as a socialite, only raising funds for her pet project, as it were, in her spare time; then returning to the mountains when this began to pall.

Data Analysis Plan

The documented data will be presented in narrative form and organized as outlined in the methodology section.

Bibliography and Research References

BOOKS

American Nurses' Association. *Priorities for Research in Nursing.* Code No. D-51 3M. Kansas City: The Association, May 1976.

Breckinridge, Mary. *Wide Neighborhoods: A Story of the*

---

3. Marquis—Who's Who, Inc., *Who Was Who in America,* Vol. 4. (St. Louis: Von Hoffman Press, Inc., 1968), p. 114.
4. Frontier Nursing Service, Inc., *Frontier Nursing Service Quarterly Bulletin.* (Wendover, Ky.: Frontier Nursing Service, Inc., 1976), p. 6.

Frontier Nursing Service. New York: Harper & Brothers, 1952.

Bullough, V. L., and Bullough, B. *The Emergence of Modern Nursing,* 2nd ed. New York: Macmillan, 1973.

Dolan, Josephine. *Nursing in Society: A Historical Perspective.* Philadelphia: W. B. Saunders, 1973.

Gatner, E. and Cordasco, F. *Research and Report Writing.* College Outline Series. New York: Barnes & Noble, 1974.

James, E. T., ed. *Notable American Women, 1607–1950: A Bibliographical Dictionary.* Vol. I. Cambridge: The Belknap Press, 1971.

Logan, Mary S. *The Part Taken by Women in American History.* New York: Arno Press, 1972.

Marquis–Who's Who, Inc. *Who was Who in America,* Vol. 4. St. Louis: Von Hoffman Press, Inc., 1968.

Maternity Center Association of New York. *Twenty Years of Nurse–Midwifery 1933–1953.* New York: Maternity Center Association, 1955.

McKeown, Robin. *Heroic Nurses.* New York: G. P. Putnam Sons, 1966.

Notter, Lucille E. *Essentials of Nursing Research.* New York: Springer, 1974.

Poole, Ernest. *Nurses on Horseback.* New York: Macmillan, 1932.

Roberts, Mary M. *American Nursing: History and Interpretations.* New York: Macmillan, 1954.

Robinson, Victor. *White Caps: The Story of Nursing.* Philadelphia: J. B. Lippincott, 1946.

Turabian, K. L. *A Manual for Writers of Term Papers, Theses and Dissertations.* Chicago: University of Chicago Press, 1972.

Wilkie, Katharine E. and Moseley, Elizabeth R. *Frontier Nurse: Mary Breckinridge.* Messner, 1969.

PERIODICALS, BULLETINS, AND PAMPHLETS

American College of Nurse–Midwives. *What Is a Nurse–Midwife?* Washington, D.C.: American College of Nurse–Midwives, 1978.

Ash, J., "District Nursing in Kentucky," *District Nurse* 5 (September 1962).

Beasley, R. "Extension of Medical Services Through Nurse Assistants." *The Journal of the Kentucky Medical Association* 67 (February 1969):101–106.

Breckinridge, Mary. "Reflections of a Septuagenerian." *British Journal of Nursing* 104 (February–March 1956).

Buck, Dorothy F. "The Nurses on Horseback Ride On." *American Journal of Nursing* 40 (September 1940):993–995.

Christy, Teresa. "The Methodology of Historical Research: A Brief Introduction." *Nursing Research* 24 (May–June 1975):189–192.

"The Frontier Nursing Service: Fifty Years of Care." *Midwives Chronicle and Nursing Notes.* May, 1975.

Frontier Nursing Service, Inc. *Frontier Nursing Service Quarterly Bulletin.* Wendover, Ky.: Frontier Nursing Service, 1976.

Hardenbrooks, Clem. "Edge of Dark Land." *Abbott Tempo* 2 (February 1964).

Holloway, James. "Frontier Nursing Service 1925–1975." *Journal of Kentucky Medical Association* 73 (September 1975):491–492.

"Mary Breckinridge." *American Journal of Nursing* 27 (March 1927):159.

"Mary Breckinridge, Nurse–Midwife." *American Journal of Nursing* 30 (March 1930):311–312.

"News About Nursing." *American Journal of Nursing* 37 (August 1937):920–921.

"News About Nursing." *American Journal of Nursing* 39 (November 1939):1385.

"Obituary." *American Journal of Nursing* 65 (July 1965):145.

"Obituary." *The New York Times* (May 17, 1965).

"Rebirth of the Midwife." *Life Magazine.* November 19, 1971.

Rochstroh, Edna C. "Enter the Nurse Midwife." (Foreword by Mary Breckinridge). *American Journal of Nursing* 27 (March 1927):159–164.

Schutt, Barbara G. "Frontier's Family Nurses." *American Journal of Nursing* 72 (May 1972):903–909.

Tirpak, Helen. "The Frontier Nursing Service: Fifty Years in the Mountains." *Nursing Outlook* 23 (May 1975): 308–310.

Walker, E. "Primex—The Family Nurse Practitioner Program." *Nursing Outlook* 20 (January 1972):28–31.

DOCTORAL DISSERTATION

Tirpak, Helen. "The Frontier Nursing Service. An Adventure in the Delivery of Health Care." Doctoral Dissertation, School of Education, University of Pittsburgh, 1972.

Appendix C

EXAMPLE OF A DESCRIPTIVE RESEARCH PROPOSAL: "LEBOYER . . . LE MAZE: IS THERE A DIFFERENCE IN INFANT TEMPERAMENT?"

By
Sharron O'Brien
(Used with Permission)

Table of Contents

Statement of the Problem
INTRODUCTION

In 1975, the publications of Dr. Frederick Leboyer's book, *Birth Without Violence,* stimulated controversy among the lay and professional communities regarding his "gentle birth" method. Since that time it has been modified to comply with the American delivery room's principles of asepsis and medical ethics. The increasing acceptability and use of the modified Leboyer method is directly attributable to the popularity of his humanistic approach to the newborn, and the research results that have failed to document any adverse effects resulting from this delivery method. Although research is currently in progress in France to determine the longterm effects of his method, there have been no substantiated reports of beneficial effects on child development and behavior resulting from Leboyer's delivery method.

This study proposes to identify whether there are differences in temperament among infants delivered by the Leboyer method and infants delivered by the LeMaze method of childbirth.

LITERATURE REVIEW

Dr. Frederick Leboyer graduated as an advanced scholar from the Faculté de Médecine in the Université de Paris in 1937. Prior to establishing his private practice, he held the rank of *chef de clinique*. By the time of his retirement in 1975, he had delivered 10,000 babies in the traditional manner and 1,000 in a manner that he philosophically describes as "gentle birth" or "birth without violence." His critics call the method foolish, dangerous and ". . . accuse him of everything from shamanism and mysticism to outright quackery." [1] His supporters, however, feel that birth without violence may contribute to human health and psychic integrity.

The innovations suggested by Leboyer are designed to assist the infant in a gradual transition from intrauterine life. This is accomplished by eliminating overstimulation of the infant's senses. The delivery room lighting is dimmed, and no one speaks above a whisper. The infant is handled gently with emphasis on not stressing the craniosacral axis, which has already been subjected to bending and pushing during travel through the birth canal. The infant is immediately placed on the mother's abdomen where the doctor and mother tenderly massage her or him while waiting for the umbilical cord to stop pulsating. Leboyer describes this delay in cutting the cord as ". . . an invitation to both the doctor and the mother to respect the baby's own life-rhythm." [2] Once the cord is severed, the infant is submerged in a bath of warm water—a brief return to a familiar environment. The baby remains in the bath until the body

---

1. Steven Englund, "Birth Without Violence," *New York Times Magazine,* December 8, 1974, p. 118.
2. Frederick Leboyer, *Birth Without Violence* (New York: Alfred A. Knopf, 1975), p. 44.

relaxation is complete—according to Leboyer, a sign that all fear has been dispelled and the pain of birth forgotten. The infant is then wrapped in layers of cotton and wool with care to cover neither the head nor hands, which are left free to move and play. The baby is then placed on its side, left to experience aloneness. This is followed by cradling and a return to mother where "lying once again on the beloved body of the mother, its ear against her heart, the baby redis-covers the familiar steady beat." [3]

Leboyer's method of childbirth was publicly described in his book, *Birth without Violence*, which was a best seller in France, and has since been translated into several languages. It appeared in the United States in 1975. As in France, Leboyer, his book, and his method stirred vehement feelings among Americans.

Professionals were shocked by his ungowned, unmasked, and ungloved conduct of childbirth. Furthermore, his choice in terming the method "birth without violence" seemed an epithet to conscientious practitioners. The reaction was im-mediate. Professionals cited his failures in sterile technique and expressed concern that the method would result in in-creased newborn infection rates and infant cold stress. Addi-tionally, Leboyer was criticized for his unscientific approach, and described as ". . . the grocerer of obstetrics and well-known for it. Moreover he has published no important scientific papers." [4]

In response to his critics, we find Dr. Leboyer stating: "they mock me by pushing my method to the extremes." [5] Yet, of his book—the only published account of his method and philosophy—written as a prose poem of sorts, it has been stated: "it reads like Dante's *Inferno* and Milton's *Paradise Regained* set side by side, a tale of horror of what Leboyer thinks most deliveries are actually like, and a poem of beauty about how they can be." [6]

---

3. Ibid., p. 101.
4. Englund, *New York Times*, p. 118.
5. Ibid.
6. Ibid., p. 113.

Despite the criticism, even professionals have been swayed by the gentle nonintervention inherent in the method and the humanistic attention to the infant that Leboyer projects. Finding these to be of value, obstetricians have accepted the requests of couples for a "gentle birth" experience; however, the method has been modified to include traditional delivery room attire. Additionally, there is variation among practitioners as to whether the mother's abdomen is draped or undraped and whether the infant's father is present in the delivery room.

Researchers have also addressed themselves to the Leboyer method in order to evaluate its safety and effects on neonatal behavior. Thus far it has been shown that no significant differences in newborn temperature, hematocrit or complications—either newborn or maternal—can be attributed to the modified gentle birth method.[7]

On the other hand, two published studies have demonstrated significant differences in neonatal behavior following delivery by a gentle birth method. One of these, based on delivery room observations of neonates, noted that infants delivered by the gentle birth method tended to be more relaxed, open their eyes more and make soft sounds. Babies delivered without gentle birth exhibited body tension, blinking, crying, sucking, and shuttering.[8]

The second study—based on observations immediately following birth, one hour after birth and following feeding 24–30 hours after birth—confirmed the researcher's hypothesis that there is an increased state of alertness in the immediate postdelivery period in infants born according to the Leboyer method.[9]

These studies are reassuring to the obstetrical practioners who have responded to the increasing public request for

7. Charlotte M. Oliver and George M. Oliver, "Gentle Birth: Its Safety and its Effect on Neonatal Behavior," *JOGN* 7 (September/October 1978):38.
8. Ibid., p. 39.
9. Alice Salter, "Birth Without Violence: A Medical Controversy," *JOGN* 27 (March/April 1978):84–88.

Leboyer childbirth experiences. However, we still have no evidence to support the suggestion that gentle birth is beneficial to the emotional health of the infant. As both studies mention, the implications of differences seen in infant behavior are yet to be investigated.

Rapoport is conducting a study in France to evaluate the long-term effects of Leboyer's delivery method on children delivered by him. Although the study is not complete, Rapoport states that the children show more interest in their environment and others; and that they ". . . use their intelligence in more positive and socially adaptive ways than other babies do." [10] Older children in the study group scored significantly higher than average when tested for "adaptivity." [11] This study when concluded and substantiated by data may support Leboyer's statement that:

> It is total error to imagine that birth without violence breeds children who are passive, weak, numb. Just the contrary.
> Birth without violence breeds children who are strong, because they are free without conflict. Free and fully awake.[12]

In summary, a review of the literature reveals articles in support, in controversy, and even providing physiological rationale for the method of childbirth purported by Dr. Frederick Leboyer. Two research projects have documented a difference in neonatal behavior following delivery by a modified Leboyer technique; they also failed to produce the devastating increase in newborn morbidity predicted by Leboyer's critics. Additionally, the literature review revealed the ease with which the Leboyer method of childbirth articulates with the theoretical framework provided by Janov's primal pain theory and Roy's adaptation model of nursing.

---

10. Englund, *New York Times,* p. 114.
11. Ibid.
12. Leboyer, *Birth without Violence,* p. 110.

THEORETICAL FRAMEWORK

The mechanics of Leboyer's gentle birth method are direct representations of his fundamental premise that babies are people with feelings and sensory abilities developed in utero and fully at work during the birth experience. He further states that the infant's perceptions are not organized and coherent and that this makes the sensations of traditional childbirth ". . . all the stronger, all the more violent, unbearable—literally maddening." [13]

His views are supported by Otto Rank, who was the first to place emphasis on the psychological importance of birth. He believed that birth represented the individual's initial encounter with anxiety, and that it would plague him throughout his life. Indeed psychiatric professionals have stressed that birth—the infant's first separation from mother —forms the core for later symptomatology.[14]

Leboyer's approach to childbirth is also supported by Arthur Janov's psychoanalytical theory of primal pain. He states that man is a creature of needs and that the needs for nourishment, love, and growth at his own pace form the infant's central reality. Janov further claims that when these needs are unmet, the individual pursues his needs symbolically thus suppressing the original pain and masking it beneath tension, neurosis and unnecessary suffering. Primal pain theory and Dr. Leboyer purport that birth profoundly influences human development and that a violent birth is the basis of lifelong psychiatric disability.[15]

According to Roy's adaptation model of nursing, man is a biopsychosocial being in constant interaction with his environment. In response to internal and external changes, man

---

13. Ibid., p. 16.
14. Bonnie Moore Randolph, "Birth and its Effects on Human Behavior," *Perspectives in Psychiatric Care* 15 (January/February/March 1977):20–26.
15. Jeffrey Gimbel and James J. Nacon, "The Psychological Basis for the Leboyer Approach to Childbirth," *JOGN* 6 (January/February 1977):11–12.

demonstrates behaviors directed toward physiologic, psychic and social integrity. His response to his changing environment is known as the process of adaptation. An adaptive response is one that maintains the integrity of the individual, and a maladaptive response is one that does not maintain integrity and is disruptive to the individual. Furthermore, the individual's ability to make an adaptive response depends on the degree of the change in his environment and the state of the individual coping with the change.

As man travels the continuum of health and illness, he will encounter adaptation problems. The goal of nursing is to assist man in his adaptation.[16]

The trend toward family-centered maternity care represents concern for the environmental changes that new parents encounter as they adapt to pregnancy, childbirth and parenting. Indeed, this philosophy of maternity care results in nursing interventions to assist adaptation toward physiologic, psychic and social integrity for the couple.

Yet, as Leboyer asks, "what about the baby?" That birth represents a change in the infant's environment is undeniable; and now we ask "is family-centered maternity care adequate in assisting the infant's adaptation toward physiologic, psychic and social integrity?"

Purpose of the Study

The purpose of this study is to answer the following question:

Is there a difference in temperament among infants delivered by a modified Leboyer method and infants delivered by the LeMaze method in a private hospital in the southeastern United States utilizing family-centered maternity care?

---

16. Sister Callista Roy, *Introduction to Nursing: An Adaptation Model* (New Jersey: Prentice-Hall, 1976), pp. 11–18.

Definition of Terms

Temperament—nine parameters of temperament will be evaluated: activity, rhythmicity, adaptability, approach, sensory threshold, intensity, mood, distractibility and persistence

Difficult temperament—that temperament in which there are 4–5 category scores on the difficult side of the mean (irregular, low in adaptability, initial withdrawal, intense, and predominantly negative mood) with at least two of these more than one standard deviation from the mean

Easy temperament—that temperament in which there are no more than two difficult category ratings, neither being greater than one standard deviation from the mean

Intermediate temperament—that temperament which falls between the criteria for easy and difficult temperament [17]

Infants—children at four months of age

Modified Leboyer Method—a method of childbirth that includes:

1. prenatal education of the expectant mother and her chosen support person—usually her husband
2. dim lighting of the delivery room
3. elimination of loud voices and noises in the delivery room
4. gentle handling of the infant
5. gentle massage of the infant by the mother and father if present
6. delay in clamping and cutting the umbilical cord until pulsations have ceased
7. placing the infant in a warm bath
8. placing the infant under a radiant warmer where routine newborn care will be accomplished (i.e., eye care, identification, etc.)
9. returning the infant to the mother for cuddling and/or breast feeding after newborn care is completed

The method is defined as modified since the delivering physician will wear the customary delivery room attire. Also,

---

17. William B. Carey, "Clinical Applications of Infant Temperament Measurements," *Behavioral Pediatrics* 81 (October 1972): 824.

husband (when present) will assist in the massage and bathing of the infant. Dr. Leboyer made no reference to the husband's role in childbirth.

LeMaze Method—a method of childbirth that includes:

1. prenatal education of the expectant mother and her chosen support person—usually her husband
2. the inclusion of the support person as a coach during the labor and delivery experience
3. the use of the psychoprophylactic method of childbirth that was publicly described by and attributed to Dr. Fernand LeMaze
4. viewing of the infant by both parents in the delivery room immediately after birth
5. placing the infant under a radiant warmer where routine newborn care will be accomplished (i.e., eye care, identification, etc.)
6. presenting the infant to the mother or father for cuddling and/or breast feeding after newborn care is completed

Family-centered maternity care—a philosophy of care that recognizes the unity and uniqueness of the family. The child's father is encouraged to participate in the intrapartum care and support of his wife and child to the extent that the couple desires. Both parents are encouraged to care for the infant at the mother's bedside with the supervision and assistance of the obstetrical nursing staff.

The Research Design

INTRODUCTION

A descriptive research design will be utilized to determine whether the independent variable of delivery method significantly influences the dependent variable of infant temperament.

SAMPLE AND SETTING

The study subjects will be selected from the three month delivery population of two obstetricians associated in private practice who perform both Leboyer and LeMaze deliveries according to the desires of the expectant parents. All infants will be delivered by these same physicians and in the same hospital, a private 500–bed facility with a 30–bed maternity unit operating under a family–centered maternity care philosophy. All infants will be the first child in the family, full-term at the time of delivery, and four months of age at the time of the study. The sample will consist of twenty infants. Ten of the infants will be delivered by a modified Leboyer method, and ten will be delivered by the LeMaze method. Any infant who develops medical complications at birth or prior to the completion of the study project will be omitted from the sample.

METHOD AND INSTRUMENT

A questionnaire will be mailed to all of the primiparous women delivered by the LeMaze and Leboyer methods in a three month period of time by a private obstetrician. Of the questionnaires returned, twenty infants meeting the sample group criteria will be randomly selected.

The questionnaire consists of seventy statements each having three choices by which the mother can describe her infant's behavior in varying situations (i.e., diapering, feeding, new foods, etc.). The tool was developed by Dr. William B. Carey for use in his private practice of pediatrics. It is directly based on the research interview of Thomas, Chess and Birch and produces similar results; however, it can be completed by the mother in approximately twenty minutes and rapidly scored. A copy of the questionnaire and written permission to use it in this study will be requested from Dr. Carey.

The most prominent technique for research on differences in infant temperament is that designed by Thomas and associates, the New York Longitudinal Study (NYLS). The NYLS, based primarily on parent interviews, was found to correlate highly with direct observations of the children.

However, application of this technique by others proves to be time consuming, tedious and open to variations in interpretation.[18]

RELIABILITY AND VALIDITY

Reliability of the questionnaire has been documented by Dr. Carey, using a test–retest method in which he noted 87–90% agreement as to rating above and below the mean.

Face and content validity of the tool will be demonstrated by submitting the questionnaire to two pediatric nurse practitioners and one pediatrician for evaluation.

Protection of Human Rights

A cover letter (see Appendix) attached to each questionnaire will introduce the purpose of the study, reassure the mothers of anonymity, and request their voluntary participation. All respondents will be provided with the telephone number of the researcher and encouraged to contact her for clarification of any aspect of the study or questionnaire.

Assumptions

Several assumptions have been made in defining the research design.

Children who demonstrate medical complications at the time of delivery or prior to the conclusion of the study will be excluded from the study based on the belief by some that even in the early months of life, temperamental differences are the result of the individual's experiences.

Based on the fact that the infants' mothers are under the care of private obstetricians, it is assumed that they will be middle class and capable of understanding and completing

---

18. William B. Carey, "A Simplified Method for Measuring Infant Temperament," *The Journal of Pediatrics* 77 (August 1970):188–189.

the written questionnaire as well as making the necessary observations of their infants.

Limitations
Mothers of the infants may be biased in completing the questionnaire either because they wish to project their baby as more socially desirable or because those mothers who elect to have a Leboyer delivery may be well acquainted with the purported benefits of this method.

Plan for Data Analysis
Characteristics of the Leboyer and LeMaze groups represent nominal data and will be expressed in percentages to allow comparison.

Table 1 Characteristics of Leboyer and LeMaze Groups

CHARACTERISTIC	LEBOYER	LEMAZE
Age of Mother:		
Mean		
Range		
Annual Income:		
Mean		
Range		
Mean Duration of Labor		
Infant Sex:		
Male		
Female		
Birth Weight:		
Mean		
Range		

Student's t test will be used to determine significant differences between the means on each of the temperament parameters as well as the total mean score for each group. The t test will be two-tailed and significance will be reported at the .05 level.

Table 2 Mean Scores of Both Groups on Temperament
Parameters

PARAMETER	LEBOYER	LEMAZE
Activity		
Rhythmicity		
Adaptability		
Approach		
Sensory Threshold		
Intensity		
Mood		
Distractibility		
Persistence		
Total Mean Score		

A table of temperament classifications will be presented,
and the data will be analyzed using Chi Square with
correction for the small sample size.

Table 3 Temperament Classifications

CLASSIFICATION	LEBOYER	LEMAZE
Difficult temperament		
Intermediate temperament		
Easy temperament		

Bibliography

Affonso, Dyanne, "The Newborn's Potential for Interaction."
JOGN 5 (November/December 1976):9–14.

Brazelton, T. B.; Scholl, M. L.; and Robey, J. S. "Visual Responses in the Newborn." *Pediatrics* 37 (February 1966):
284–290.

Carey, William B. "A Simplified Method for Measuring Infant Temperament." *Journal of Pediatrics* 77 (August
1970):188–194.

Carey, William B. "Clinical Applications of Infant Temperament Measurements." *Behavioral Pediatrics* 81 (October 1972):823–827.

Davies, Rachel; Hogan, Margo; and Russell, Kate. "A Sensitive Approach to Childbirth." *Nursing Times* 74 (February 9, 1978):222–224.

Englund, Steven. "Birth Without Violence." *New York Times Magazine,* December 8, 1974, pp. 113–118.

Gimbel, Jeffrey, and Nacon, James J. "The Physiological Basis for the Leboyer Approach to Childbirth." *JOGN* 6 (January/February 1977):11–15.

Klaus, M. et al. "Maternal Attachment: Importance of the First Postpartum Days. *New England Journal of Medicine* 286 (March 1972):460–463.

Leboyer, Frederick. *Birth without Violence.* New York: Alfred A. Knopf, 1975.

Oliver, Charlotte M., and Oliver, George M. "Gentle Birth: Its Safety and Its Effect on Neonatal Behavior." *JOGN* (September/October 1978):35–40.

Phillips, Celeste R. "The Essence of Birth without Violence." *The American Journal of Maternal Child Nursing* 6 (May/June 1976):162–163.

Randolph, Bonnie Moore. "Birth and Its Effects on Human Behavior." *Perspectives in Psychiatric Care* 15 (January/February/March 1977):20–26.

Roy, Callista, Sister. *Introduction to Nursing: An Adaptation Model.* New Jersey: Prentice-Hall, 1976.

Salter, Alice. "Birth without Violence: A Medical Controversy." *JOGN* 27 (March/April 1978):84–88.

Appendix:
QUESTIONNAIRE COVER LETTER

Date

Dear Mrs. ———:

I am a student nurse conducting a research project in cooperation with your obstetrician, Dr. ———.

The purpose of this study is to investigate infant temperament.

I would greatly appreciate your participation in this study. Realizing that your time is limited, I am using a short questionnaire that takes about twenty minutes to fill in.

I have enclosed a stamped, self-addressed envelope and would appreciate your filling out the questionnaire and returning it to me as soon as possible.

Although mothers who assist in this study will remain anonymous, I encourage you to call me about the study itself or the questionnaire if you have any questions. I would also be happy to share the results of the study with you when it is completed.

Thank you for your assistance, and congratulations on the birth of your first baby!

Sincerely,

Sharron O'Brien
Phone: ———
Address: ———

Appendix D

EXAMPLE OF AN EXPERIMENTAL RESEARCH PROPOSAL: "THE PHYSIOLOGIC EFFECTS OF KINETIC NURSING ON PARTIAL PRESSURES AND ACIDITY IN IMMOBILIZED PATIENTS' ARTERIAL BLOOD GAS VALUES"

By
Kathy L. Green
(Used with Permission)

Table of Contents

Statement of the Problem

The hazards of immobility on all of our bodily systems are all too apparent to those of us in the health professions. It is quite obvious that movement is by far the most important activity for which our organism is equipped. The human body, unlike an inanimate machine, improves with use and deteriorates with lack of use. It stands to reason that in man there must be a minimal degree of activity below which serious degeneration arises.[1] In the immobilized patient, this minimal degree of activity is lacking, thus predisposing the patient to succumbing to the hazards of immobility, especially those life-threatening hazards affecting the respiratory system. Immobilized patients nursed on a traditional hospital bed, a Stryker frame, or a circ-o-electric bed, are usually turned at two hour intervals, but are virtually immobile in between these turns. This method of care seems to be self-defeating, as respiratory complications can develop in a relatively short period of time from stasis of

---

1. F. X. Keane, "Kinetic Nursing," unpublished article, p. 1.

pulmonary secretions. It is this researcher's opinion that the way to avoid these respiratory complications would be to nurse the patient kinetically by use of the Roto-Rest Bed. The constant side-to-side motion provided by this bed helps to maintain the body's homeostatic mechanisms, thus preventing respiratory deterioration. For this reason, the effect of kinetic nursing on the immobilized patients' respiratory status will be determined through the analysis of a series of arterial blood gas values.

Literature Review

The hazards of immobility on normal men were first described in 1948 in the classic studies of Deitrick, Whedon, and Shorr. They studied four men before, during, and following a prolonged period of bedrest. Activity in bed was standardized by immobilization of the pelvic girdle and legs in plastic casts. They reported the effects of immobilization on all of the bodily systems. The effects on the respiratory system itself did not prove to be remarkable. The vital capacity, ventilation at rest, and maximum ventilation capacity showed no significant changes during immobilization. It was of interest that, although maximum ventilation capacity was unimpaired during immobilization, more subjective effort seemed to be required to achieve the same result as was obtained during the control period.[2]

In 1949, these same researchers studied the modification of the effects of immobilization by the use of an oscillating bed. The Sanders oscillating bed, which effects postural changes by rotating the patient in a head-to-foot motion, was used in the study. Three men were studied in these beds before, during, and following a five-week period of immobilization in plaster casts. These three subjects had all taken

---

2. John E. Deitrick, Donald Whedon, and Ephraim Shorr, "Effects of Immobilization Upon Various Metabolic and Physiologic Functions of Normal Men," *American Journal of Medicine* 4 (January 1948):4, 22.

part in the immobilization experiment of 1948 on traditional hospital beds. The effects on the respiratory system in this second study were also unremarkable. Shifts in the position of the diaphragm occurred due to the head-to-foot oscillation of the bed. Despite these shifts, minute ventilation at rest was not greater during oscillation than in the stationary horizontal position.[3] Arterial blood gas analyses were not done in either of these studies.

The effects of immobility on respiratory function were not given much further attention until 1967. At this time it was stated that three physiologic effects on the respiratory system might occur as a result of immobility. The first one was a decrease in respiratory movement. Chest cage expansion could be limited by poor body positioning leading to compression of the thorax. Also, movement of the chest could be hindered by a diminution of muscle power and coordination due to muscle disuse. This decreased lung expansion would hinder the normal efficient and effective ventilation of air in and out of the lung tissue.

The second physiologic effect of immobility was stasis of secretions. Prolonged immobility was found to cause stasis and pooling of secretions. Due to the stasis, patients would be prone to developing hypostatic pneumonia.

The third physiologic effect of immobility was an oxygen–carbon dioxide imbalance. A decrease in respiratory movement coupled with stasis of secretions would create limited diffusion of oxygen and carbon dioxide via the alveolar and capillary membranes, and thus would alter arterial blood gas values.[4]

Keane, in 1967, reported a decreased incidence of respiratory complications when treating an immobilized patient on the Roto-Rest Bed. He also observed that patients

---

3. Donald Whedon, John E. Deitrick, and Ephraim Shorr, "Modification of the Effects of Immobilization Upon Metabolic and Physiologic Functions of Normal Men by the Use of an Oscillating Bed," *American Journal of Medicine* 8 (June 1949):685.
4. Lida F. Thompson, "The Hazards of Immobility: Effects on Respiratory Function," *American Journal of Nursing* 67 (April 1967): 3–4.

who had already developed pulmonary stasis improved rapidly when treated kinetically.[5]

In 1978, three physicians reported a case study of a 48 year old male suffering from a gunshot wound to the right axilla, who subsequently developed acute hypoxemic hypocarbic respiratory failure. He was treated on the Roto-Rest Bed with the use of combined modalities such as IMV, PEEP, and augmentation of cardiovascular function. By 18 hours after admission to the intensive care unit and implementation of the above modalities, the patient's PaO_2 (partial pressure of oxygen in the arterial blood) and cardiac output had come from dangerously low limits to registering within normal limits. In these authors' four years experience in treating this type of injury, they had never seen such a rapid resolution. They concluded that the addition of a new variable, the Roto-Rest Bed, could have played a role in the rapid resolution. They recommended that the Roto-Rest Bed should be further evaluated as a simple mechanical approach to a difficult clinical problem.[6]

In conclusion, the review of the literature gives some insight into the effects of immobility on the patient's respiratory status. Virtually no information on kinetic nursing's effect on the patient's respiratory status is available. To date, no studies have been done concerning the effects of kinesis or akinesis on the patient's arterial blood gas values. Thus, the variables to be tested in this study have never been tested before, which helps substantiate this researcher's concern.

Conceptual Framework

The story of kinetic nursing is the story of a unique man and his dream. The man is Dr. F. X. Keane, and his

---

5. F. X. Keane, "Roto-Rest," *British Medical Journal* 16 (September 1967):3–4.
6. Lawrence Schimmel, Joseph M. Civetta, Robert Kirby, "Treatment of Unilateral Pulmonary Contusion by a New Mechanical Method to Influence Pulmonary Perfusion," *Journal of Critical Care Medicine* (November–December 1977):206.

dream was to eliminate the devastating morbidity and mortality associated with the complications accruing from immobility.

As a child he watched his father, a physician, cope with the ravages of infections and diseases with little else except his common sense. One of his most clever methods of treatment was the sewing of yarn balls to the bed shirts of pneumonia victims. Whenever the patient would lie in one position for more than a few minutes, he would become very uncomfortable and turn. Therefore, Dr. Keane Sr. was able to institute postural drainage and treat pneumonia by stimulating the patient to turn 24 hours a day. It was this form of medical science that Dr. Keane Jr. applied to the design of his new concept of kinetic nursing.[7]

The solution to the complex problems of immobility became very apparent to him. The treatment for akinesis, or lack of motion, should be a form of motion or kinesis. Thus, the concept of kinetic nursing was born and the design of the Keane Roto-Rest Bed was conceived. It was designed to introduce automation into the nursing of immobilized patients. Dr. Keane defines kinetic nursing as "the automatic and continuous turning of a patient equally from side-to-side, in a given posture, through a maximum excursion of 124 degrees at a minimum rate of 124 degrees in 4.5 minutes." [8]

This concept of kinetic nursing was based on his study of motion. He realized that movement or activity was of such fundamental importance to man that even during sleep the normal healthy adult must, and does, turn or change position approximately every 11.6 minutes. He termed this essential activity the minimum physiological mobility requirement.[9]

The Roto-Rest Bed has the same proportions of the usual hospital bed and is electrically operated by a silent 1/7

---

7. B. A. Green, "Kinetic Nursing for Spinal Cord Injuries," *Paraplegia Life* (January–February 1976), p. 1.

8. F. X. Keane, "Kinetic Nursing," p. 4.

9. Ibid., p. 1.

horsepower motor that uses power equal to that of a 60-watt light bulb. The entire bed is made of hatches that may be opened from underneath, enabling the nurse to give back care or other routine nursing care. Each hatch is covered with a cushion its own size on which the patient lies. The patient is centered on the bed, and then side packs are positioned snugly to hold the body in alignment. Knee and shoulder packs overlie these bony parts and act to prevent the patient from falling out of bed.[10] The bed may be manually manipulated to any of nine locked positions and can be positioned in Trendelenburg or reverse Trendelenburg as well.

Purpose of the Study

The purpose of this study will be to test the following hypothesis: In the neurosurgical intensive care unit at a large county hospital, there will be no significant change in immobilized patients' arterial blood gas values when the Roto-Rest Bed is temporarily stopped.

Definition of Terms

Traditional hospital bed   An electrically operated bed that has a control that allows the patient to raise or lower the head and knee gatches.

Immobilized patients   Newly admitted patients of any age group confined to total bedrest on the Roto-Rest Bed as the result of a head injury, spinal cord injury, or multiple traumatic injuries.

Arterial blood gas values   A laboratory study of arterial blood samples for the purpose of measuring oxygen and carbon dioxide levels, and hydrogen ion concentration. The blood gas values will act as the dependent variable in this study.

---

10. Lorraine Valentin, "Kinetic Nursing and the Roto-Rest Bed, *Orthopedic Nurses' Association Journal* 4 (March 1977):63.

PaO₂ Partial pressure (P) of oxygen (O_2) in the arterial blood (a). Normal range of values 80–100 mm Hg.
PaCO₂ Partial pressure (P) of carbon dioxide (CO_2) in the arterial blood (a). Normal range of values 35–45 mm Hg.
pH A measure of the acidity or alkalinity in the blood by measuring the hydrogen ion concentration. Normal values 7.35–7.45.

Roto-Rest Bed An electrically operated bed that constantly rotates the patient slowly from side-to-side. The complete cycle rotates the patient 124 degrees in 4.5 minutes.

Temporarily stopped The bed will be rotating until the experimenter turns it off, leaving the patient in a fixed horizontal position for a period of exactly 2 hours. After that 2 hour period of time the bed will be started again.

Kinetic nursing This phrase will be used to refer to any immobilized patient being treated on the Roto-Rest Bed.

Kinesis Motion
Akinesis Lack of motion

Methodology
RESEARCH DESIGN

To study the effect of kinetic nursing on arterial blood gas values, an experimental design will be used. Physiological measures will be used to collect data from the subjects.

SAMPLING PROCEDURES

The target population will consist of patients in the neurosurgical intensive care unit at a large county hospital being treated on the Roto-Rest Bed. A convenience (non-probability) sample will be used in this study. The sample will include the first 10 patients admitted to the neurosurgical intensive care unit as a result of a head injury, a spinal cord injury or multiple traumatic injuries, as of January 1, 1979. Only those patients treated on the Roto-Rest Bed will be included in this study. The blood samples for study will be obtained from these first 10 patients regardless of their age, sex, stage of illness, or other extraneous variables.

DATA COLLECTION

The data to be collected will be quantitative in nature. It will be obtained by drawing arterial blood samples from the arterial line and sending them to the lab for blood gas analysis. The patients will act as their own controls. The procedure will be as follows:

Step 1. The first arterial blood gas sample will be drawn after the patient has been allowed to rotate on the Roto-Rest Bed for an uninterrupted 2 hour period. The bed will be stopped and locked in position after this 2 hour period, and the blood gas will be drawn immediately. This will constitute the premeasure (T_1) and will be considered to reflect the effects of kinesis on the arterial blood gas values.

Step 2. The bed will be kept in this locked horizontal position for exactly 2 hours. At the end of that period of time another arterial blood gas sample will be obtained. This sample will constitute the first postmeasure (T_2) and will be considered to reflect the effects of akinesis on the arterial blood gas values.

Step 3. After the second sample is obtained the bed will be started again and will assume its normal rotation. The patient will be allowed to rotate for an uninterrupted 2 hour period. The bed will then be stopped again so that the third and final arterial blood gas can be immediately drawn. This sample will constitute the second postmeasure (T_3) and will be considered to reflect the effects of kinesis on the arterial blood gas values.

Step 4. The bed will be restarted once again as the study of this patient will have been completed.

The elements to be examined in this study will include the PaO_2, $PaCO_2$, and pH. The effect of kinesis or akinesis on these parameters will be determined.

PILOT STUDY

This protocol for analyzing the arterial blood gas values at intervals was tested prior to the final writing of this proposal. Two spinal cord injured patients on the Roto-Rest Bed were the subjects in the pilot study. An arterial blood gas was drawn after the bed had been rotating for one hour. Another was drawn after the bed had been in a fixed horizontal position for one hour and the final sample was drawn after the bed had been rotating again for one hour. There were no changes in the PaO_2, $PaCO_2$, or pH, during the period of kinesis or akinesis. This led the researcher to extend the time intervals to 2-hour intervals as discussed in this proposal under data collection.

LIMITATIONS

There will be limitations in projecting the results to the population due to the small sample size and the non-probability sampling procedure.

ETHICAL CONSIDERATIONS

Each subject will receive an explanation about the purpose and nature of the study. Subjects will be told that the information obtained will be used by the physicians to evaluate when they can be safely transferred to a traditional hospital bed. Confidentiality will be maintained. The subject will not at any time be exposed to physical harm due to this research. Since this series of blood gas analyses has been incorporated into the written protocol for any patient treated kinetically in the neurosurgical intensive care unit in which this study will be conducted, the costs to the patient will not exceed the normal costs accrued during this stage of treatment.

Data Analysis

The data for each of the dependent measures (PaO_2, $PaCO_2$, and pH) will be analyzed by using separate one-way repeated analysis of variance measures (F tests). Analysis of variance will be used because there will be more than 2 measurement points. Repeated measures will be used because the subjects will be used as their own control. The data being analyzed will relate to time and measurement (i.e. the 3 time periods and the 3 parameters being measured). The level of significance for rejection of the null hypothesis will be at the .05 level.

The following tables will be used:

Table 1 Means for Blood Gas Values by Time Periods

BLOOD GAS VALUES	TIME PERIODS *		
	T_1	T_2	T_3
PaO_2			
$PaCO_2$			
pH			

* Time Periods
  T_1 = premeasure (rotating bed)
  T_2 = postmeasure (bed stabilized)
  T_3 = postmeasure (bed rotating)

Table 2 Analysis of Variance Design for Each Different Measure by Study Subjects

SUBJECT NO.	TIME PERIODS		
	T_1	T_2	T_3
S_1	S_1T_1	S_1T_2	S_1T_3
S_2	S_2T_1	S_2T_2	S_2T_3
S_3	S_3T_1	S_3T_2	S_3T_3
S_4	S_4T_1	S_4T_2	S_4T_3
S_5	S_5T_1	S_5T_2	S_5T_3
S_6	S_6T_1	S_6T_2	S_6T_3
S_7	S_7T_1	S_7T_2	S_7T_3
S_8	S_8T_1	S_8T_2	S_8T_3
S_9	S_9T_1	S_9T_2	S_9T_3
S_{10}	$S_{10}T_1$	$S_{10}T_2$	$S_{10}T_3$

Table 3 Source of Variation Table

	SS	DF	MS	F	P
Source					
Subjects					
Time					
Subjects × Time					

Bibliography

Brink, Pamela J., and Ward, Marilynn J. *Basic Steps in Planning Nursing Research.* North Scituate, Mass.: Duxbury Press, 1978.

Deitrick, John E., Whedon, Donald, and Shorr, Ephraim. "Effects of Immobilization Upon Various Metabolic and Physiologic Functions of Normal Men." *American Journal of Medicine* 8 (January 1948):3–34.

Ferguson, George A. *Statistical Analysis in Psychology and Education.* New York: McGraw-Hill, 1976.

Green, B. A. "Kinetic Nursing for Spinal Cord Injuries." *Paraplegia Life* (January–February 1976):1–5.

Keane, F. X. "Kinetic Nursing." Unpublished article: 1–4.

Keane, F. X. "Roto–Rest." *British Medical Journal* 16 (September 1967):731–733.

Miller, Benjamin F., and Keane, Claire. *Encyclopedia and Dictionary of Medicine, Nursing, and Allied Health.* Philadelphia: W. B. Saunders, 1978.

Schimmel, Lawrence, Civetta, Joseph, and Kirby, Robert R. "Treatment of Unilateral Pulmonary Contusion by a New Mechanical Method to Influence Pulmonary Perfusion." *Journal of Critical Care Medicine* (November–December 1977):206–207.

Thompson, Lida F. "The Hazards of Immobility: Effects on Respiratory Function." *American Journal of Nursing* 67 (April 1967):1–17.

Valentin, Lorraine. "Kinetic Nursing and the Roto-Rest Bed." *Orthopedic Nurses' Association Journal* 4 (March 1977):62–65.

Whedon, Donald, Deitrick, John E., Shorr, Ephraim. "Modification of the Effects of Immobilization Upon Metabolic and Physiologic Functions of Normal Men by the Use of an Oscillating Bed." *American Journal of Medicine* 8 (June 1949):684–710.

Appendix E

EXAMPLE OF A RESEARCH REPORT: "THE PHYSIOLOGIC EFFECTS OF KINETIC NURSING ON PARTIAL PRESSURES AND ACIDITY IN IMMOBILIZED PATIENTS' ARTERIAL BLOOD GAS VALUES"

By
Kathy L. Green
(Used with Permission)

Table of Contents

List of Tables

Introduction

STATEMENT OF THE PROBLEM

The hazards of immobility on all of our bodily systems are all too apparent to those of us in the health professions.

It is quite obvious that movement is by far the most important activity for which our organism is equipped. The human body, unlike an inanimate machine, improves with use and deteriorates with lack of use. It stands to reason that in man there must be a minimal degree of activity below which serious degeneration arises.[1] In the immobilized patient, this minimal degree of activity is lacking, thus predisposing the patient to succumbing to the hazards of immobility, especially those life threatening hazards affecting the respiratory system. Immobilized patients nursed on a traditional hospital bed, a Stryker frame, or a circ-o-electric bed, are usually turned at two hour intervals, but are virtually immobile in between these turns. This method of care seems to be self-defeating, as respiratory complications can develop in a relatively short period of time from stasis of pulmonary secretions. It is this researcher's opinion that the way to avoid these respiratory complications would be to nurse the patient kinetically by use of the Roto-Rest Bed. The constant side-to-side motion provided by this bed helps to maintain the body's homeostatic mechanisms, thus preventing respiratory deterioration. For this reason, the effect of kinetic nursing on the immobilized patients' respiratory status was determined through the analysis of a series of arterial blood gas values.

LITERATURE REVIEW

The hazards of immobility on normal men were first described in 1948 in the classic studies of Deitrick, Whedon, and Shorr. They studied four men before, during, and following a prolonged period of bedrest. Activity in bed was standardized by immobilization of the pelvic girdle and legs in plastic casts. They reported the effects of immobilization on all of the bodily systems. The effects on the respiratory system itself did not prove to be remarkable. The vital capacity, ventilation at rest, and maximum ventilation capac-

---

1. F. X. Keane, "Kinetic Nursing," unpublished article, p. 1.

ity showed no significant changes during immobilization. It
was of interest that, although maximum ventilation capacity
was unimpaired during immobilization, more subjective
effort seemed to be required to achieve the same result as
was obtained during the control period.[2]

In 1949, these same researchers studied the modification
of the effects of immobilization by the use of an oscillating
bed. The Sanders oscillating bed, which effects postural
changes by rotating the patient in a head-to-foot motion, was
used in the study. Three men were studied in these beds
before, during, and following a five-week period of immobilization in plaster casts. These three subjects had all taken
part in the immobilization experiment of 1948 on traditional
hospital beds. The effects on the respiratory system in this
second study were also unremarkable. Shifts in the position of
the diaphragm occurred due to the head-to-foot oscillation of
the bed. Despite these shifts, minute ventilation at rest was
not greater during oscillation than in the stationary horizontal
position.[3] Arterial blood gas analyses were not done in either
of these studies.

The effects of immobility on respiratory function were
not given much further attention until 1967. At this time
it was stated that three physiologic effects on the respiratory
system might occur as a result of immobility. The first one
was a decrease in respiratory movement. Chest cage expansion could be limited by poor body positioning, leading to
compression of the thorax. Also, movement of the chest could
be hindered by a diminution of muscle power and coordination due to muscle disuse. This decreased lung expansion

---

2. John E. Dietrick, Donald Whedon, and Ephraim Shorr, "Effects of
   Immobilization upon Various Metabolic and Physiologic Functions of Normal Men," *American Journal of Medicine* 4 (January
   1948):4, 22.
3. Donald Whedon, John E. Deitrick, and Ephraim Shorr, "Modification of the Effects of Immobilization Upon Metabolic and Physiologic Functions of Normal Men by the Use of an Oscillating
   Bed," *American Journal of Medicine* 8 (June 1949):685.

would hinder the normal efficient and effective ventilation of air in and out of the lung tissue.

The second physiologic effect of immobility was stasis of secretions. Prolonged immobility was found to cause stasis and pooling of secretions. Due to the stasis, patients would be prone to developing hypostatic pneumonia.

The third physiologic effect of immobility was an oxygen-carbon dioxide imbalance. A decrease in respiratory movement coupled with stasis of secretions would create limited diffusion of oxygen and carbon dioxide via the alveolar and capillary membranes, and thus would alter arterial blood gas values.[4]

Keane, in 1967, reported a decreased incidence of respiratory complications when treating immobilized patients on the Roto-Rest Bed. He also observed that patients who had already developed pulmonary stasis improved rapidly when treated kinetically.[5]

In 1978, three physicians reported a case study of a 48 year old male suffering from a gunshot wound to the right axilla, who subsequently developed acute hypoxemic hypocarbic respiratory failure. He was treated on the Roto-Rest Bed with the use of combined modalities such as IMV, PEEP, and augmentation of cardio-vascular function. By 18 hours after admission to the intensive care unit and implementation of the above modalities, the patient's PaO_2 (partial pressure of oxygen in the arterial blood) and cardiac output had come from dangerously low limits to registering within normal limits. In these authors' four years experience in treating this type of injury, they had never seen such a rapid resolution. They concluded that the addition of a new variable, the Roto-Rest Bed, could have played a role in the

---

4. Lida F. Thompson, "The Hazards of Immobility: Effects on Respiratory Function," *American Journal of Nursing* 67 (April 1967): 3–4.

5. F. X. Keane, "Roto-Rest," *British Medical Journal* 16 (September 1967), pp. 3–4.

rapid resolution. They recommended that the Roto-Rest Bed should be further evaluated as a simple mechanical approach to a difficult clinical problem.[6]

In conclusion, the review of the literature gave some insight into the effects of immobility on the patient's respiratory status. Very little information on kinetic nursing's effect on the patient's respiratory status was available. Prior to this study no studies had been done concerning the effects of kinesis or akinesis on the patient's arterial blood gas values. Thus, the variables being tested in this study have never been tested before, which helped to substantiate this researcher's concern.

CONCEPTUAL FRAMEWORK

The story of kinetic nursing is the story of a unique man and his dream. The man is Dr. F. X. Keane, and his dream was to eliminate the devastating morbidity and mortality associated with the complications accruing from immobility.

As a child he watched his father, a physician, cope with the ravages of infections and diseases with little else except his common sense. One of his most clever methods of treatment was the sewing of yarn balls to the bed shirts of pneumonia victims. Whenever the patient would lie in one position for more than a few minutes, he would become very uncomfortable and turn. Therefore, Dr. Keane Sr. was able to institute postural drainage and treat pneumonia by stimulating the patient to turn 24 hours a day. It was this form of medical science that Dr. Keane Jr. applied to the design of his new concept of kinetic nursing.[7]

---

6. Lawrence Schimmel, Joseph M. Civetta, Robert Kirby, "Treatment of Unilateral Pulmonary Contusion by a New Mechanical Method to Influence Pulmonary Perfusion," *Journal of Critical Care Medicine* (November–December 1977):206.
7. B. A. Green, "Kinetic Nursing for Spinal Cord Injuries," *Paraplegia Life* (January–February 1976):1.

The solution to the complex problems of immobility became very apparent to him. The treatment for akinesis, or lack of motion, should be a form of motion or kinesis. Thus, the concept of kinetic nursing was born and the design of the Keane Roto-Rest Bed was conceived. It was designed to introduce automation into the nursing of immobilized patients. Dr. Keane defines kinetic nursing as "the automatic and continuous turning of a patient equally from side-to-side, in a given posture, through a maximum excursion of 124 degrees at a minimum rate of 124 degrees in 4.5 minutes." [8]

This concept of kinetic nursing was based on his study of motion. He realized that movement or activity was of such fundamental importance to man that even during sleep the normal healthy adult must, and does, turn or change position approximately every 11.6 minutes. He termed this essential activity the minimum physiological mobility requirement.[9]

The Roto-Rest Bed has the same proportions of the usual hospital bed and is electrically operated by a silent 1/7 horsepower motor which uses power equal to that of a 60 watt light bulb. The entire bed is made of hatches that may be opened from underneath, enabling the nurse to give back care or other routine nursing care. Each hatch is covered with a cushion its own size on which the patient lies. The patient is centered on the bed and then side packs are positioned snugly to hold the body in alignment. Knee and shoulder packs overlie these bony parts and act to prevent the patient from falling out of bed.[10] The bed may be manually manipulated to any of nine locked positions and can be positioned in either Trendelenburg or reverse Trendelenburg.

---

8. F. X. Keane, "Kinetic Nursing," p. 4.
9. Ibid., p. 1.
10. Lorraine Valentin, "Kinetic Nursing and the Roto-Rest Bed," *Orthopedic Nurses' Association Journal* 4 (March 1977):63.

PURPOSE OF THE STUDY

The purpose of this study was to test the following hypothesis: In the neurosurgical intensive care unit at a large county hospital there will be no significant change in immobilized patients' arterial blood gas values when the Roto-Rest Bed is temporarily stopped.

DEFINITION OF TERMS

Traditional Hospital Bed   An electrically operated bed that has a control which allows the patient to raise or lower the head and knee gatches.

Immobilized Patients   Newly admitted patients of any age group confined to total bedrest on the Roto-Rest Bed as the result of a head injury, spinal cord injury, or multiple traumatic injuries.

Arterial Blood Gas Values   A laboratory study of arterial blood samples for the purpose of measuring oxygen and carbon dioxide levels, and hydrogen ion concentration. The blood gas values acted as the dependent variable in this study.

PaO_2   Partial pressure (P) of oxygen (O_2) in the arterial blood (a). Normal range of values 80–100 mm Hg.

$PaCO_2$ Partial pressure (P) of carbon dioxide (CO_2) in the arterial blood (a). Normal range of values 35–45 mm Hg.

pH: A measure of acidity or alkalinity in the blood by measuring the hydrogen ion concentration. Normal values 7.35–7.45.

Roto-Rest Bed   An electrically operated bed that constantly rotates the patient slowly from side-to-side. The complete cycle rotates the patient 124 degrees in 4.5 minutes.

Temporarily Stopped   The bed rotated until the experimenter manipulated the independent variable by turning it off, leaving the patient in a fixed horizontal position for a period of exactly 2 hours. After that 2 hour period of time the bed was started again.

Kinetic Nursing   This phrase was used to refer to any immobilized patient being treated on the Roto-Rest Bed.

Kinesis   Motion

Akinesis   Lack of motion

Methodology

RESEARCH DESIGN

To study the effect of kinetic nursing on arterial blood gas values, an experimental design was used. Physiological measures were used to collect data from the subjects.

STUDY SUBJECTS

The target population consisted of patients in the neurosurgical intensive care unit at a large county hospital being treated on the Roto-Rest Bed. A convenience (nonprobability) sample was used in the study. The sample included the first ten patients admitted to the neurosurgical intensive care unit as a result of a head injury, a spinal cord injury, or multiple traumatic injuries as of January 1, 1979. Only those patients treated on the Roto-Rest Bed were included in this study. The blood samples for study were obtained from these first ten patients regardless of their age, sex, stage of illness, or other extraneous variables.

DATA COLLECTION

The data to be collected were quantitative in nature. They were obtained by drawing arterial blood samples from the arterial line and sending them to the lab for blood gas analyses. The patients acted as their own controls. The procedure was as follows:

Step 1. The first arterial blood gas sample was drawn after the patient had been allowed to rotate on the Roto-Rest Bed for an uninterrupted 2 hour period. The bed was stopped and locked in position after this 2 hour period, and the blood gas was drawn immediately. This constituted the premeasure (T_1) and was considered to reflect the effects of kinesis on the arterial blood gas values.

Step 2. The bed was kept in this locked horizontal position for exactly 2 hours. At the end of that period of time another arterial blood gas sample was obtained. This sample constituted the first postmeasure (T_2) and was considered to reflect the effects of akinesis on the arterial blood gas values.

Step 3. After the second sample was obtained the bed was started again and assumed its normal rotation. The patient was allowed to rotate for an uninterrupted 2 hour period. The bed was stopped again so that the third and final arterial blood gas could be immediately drawn. This sample constituted the second postmeasure (T_3) and was considered to reflect the effects of kinesis on the arterial blood gas values.

Step 4. The bed was restarted once again as the study of this patient was completed.

The elements examined in this study included the PaO_2, $PaCO_2$ and pH. The effect of kinesis or akinesis on these parameters was determined.

PILOT STUDY

The protocol for analyzing the arterial blood gas values at hourly intervals was initially tested during the planning phase of the study. Two spinal cord injured patients on the Roto-Rest Bed were the subjects in the pilot study. An arterial blood gas was drawn after the bed had been rotating for one hour. Another was drawn after the bed had been in a fixed horizontal position for one hour and the final sample was drawn after the bed had been rotating again for one hour. There were no changes in the PaO_2, $PaCO_2$, or pH, during the periods of kinesis or akinesis. This led the researcher to extend the time to 2 hour intervals as discussed under data collection.

ETHICAL CONSIDERATIONS

Each subject received an explanation about the purpose and nature of the study. Subjects were told that the information obtained would be used by the physicians to evaluate when they could be safely transferred to a traditional hospital bed, and that confidentiality would be maintained. The patients were not at any time exposed to physical harm due to this research. Since this series of blood gas analyses had been incorporated into the written protocol for any patient treated kinetically in the neurosurgical intensive care unit in which this study was conducted, the cost to the patient did not exceed the costs normally accrued during this stage of treatment.

ANALYSIS OF THE DATA

The data for each of the dependent measures (PaO_2, $PaCO_2$, and pH) were analyzed by using separate one-way repeated analysis of variance measures (F tests). Analysis of variance was used because there were more than 2 measurement points. Repeated measures were used because the subjects acted as their own control. The major factors being tested were time and measurement (i.e. the 3 time periods and the 3 parameters being measured). The level of significance for rejection of the null hypothesis was set at the .05 level.

Findings

All ten subjects in the convenience sample were males. The age range was from 17–35 years of age. Eight patients were admitted with spinal cord injuries and the other 2 were admitted due to multiple trauma. No patient had a history of any preexisting pulmonary disease entities.

There were no significant differences found across time for any of the three dependent measures. The means for the pH and $PaCO_2$ were within normal limits across the 3 time periods, with a gradual compensatory increase noted between

Table 1 Means for Blood Gas Values by Time Periods

BLOOD GAS VALUES	TIME PERIODS *		
	T_1	T_2	T_3
PaO_2	103.0	100.9	101.1
$PaCO_2$	37.8	38.3	39.6
pH	7.40	7.41	7.42

* Time Periods
T_1 = premeasure (rotating bed)
T_2 = postmeasure (bed stabilized)
T_3 = postmeasure (bed rotating)

each dependent measure across time. The means for the PaO_2 were above normal during T_1 and T_3 (see Table 1).

The analysis of variance was not significant for any of the 3 dependent measures across time. The F ratio for the PaO_2 was < 1 (see Table 2).

The F ratio for the $PaCO_2$ was found to be 2.33 (see Table 3).

The F ratio for the pH was found to be 2.0 (see Table 4).

Due to the lack of statistical significance the data did not allow the researcher to reject the null hypothesis.

Discussion
INTERPRETATION OF FINDINGS

Unlike the traditional approaches to the evaluation of the effects of immobility on the patients' respiratory system, this study examined the effects of kinetic nursing on the

Table 2 Analysis of Variance for PaO_2 Measure Across Time

	SS	DF	MS	F	P
Time	26.87	2	13.43	< 1	ns
Subjects × Time	845.80	18	46.99		

Table 3 Analysis of Variance for $PaCO_2$ Measure Across Time

	SS	DF	MS	F	P
Time	17.27	2	8.63	2.33	ns
Subjects × Time	66.73	18	3.71		

patients' arterial blood gases by testing the following hypothesis: In the neurosurgical intensive care unit at a large county hospital there will be no significant change in immobilized patients' arterial blood gas values when the Roto-Rest Bed is temporarily stopped. The study consisted of a convenience sample of 10 neurological patients ranging from 17 to 35 years of age who were treated on the Roto-Rest Bed. A series of 3 arterial blood gases were obtained at specified time intervals. The PaO_2, and $PaCO_2$, and pH were examined to determine if alternating periods of kinesis and akinesis had any effect on these dependent measures. The findings pointed to a lack of statistical significance and the null hypothesis was supported. The nonprobability sampling procedure precludes inferring the study results to the target population. Limitations of the study include the small sample size and the limited age range of the study subjects.

Table 4 Analysis of Variance for pH Measure Across Time

	SS	DF	MS	F	P
Time	.0016	2	.0008	2.0	ns
Subjects × Time	.0080	18	.0004		

RECOMMENDATIONS FOR FUTURE STUDY

Clearly, the study raises questions for future research in spite of the fact that the study showed no statistical significance. Replication of the study, assuming certain modifications, could result in clinical significance. As a result of many positive clinical experiences in using the Roto-Rest

Bed for immobilized patients, this researcher feels that the study should be repeated using a modified format. Suggestions for future studies are as follows:

(A) Arterial blood gas values (PaO_2, $PaCO_2$, and pH) would be analyzed for a group of kinetically nursed patients. Two separate samples would be obtained from each patient which would be reflective of 1) a two hour period of kinesis and 2) a two hour period of akinesis. These samples would be obtained 24 hours prior to transfer to a traditional hospital bed. Twenty-four and 48 hours posttransfer to a traditional hospital bed, samples for blood gas analyses would be obtained to determine if any significant changes in the patients' respiratory status had occurred as a result of the cessation of kinetic nursing.

(B) Arterial blood gas values would be analyzed in a group of kinetically nursed patients utilizing various extreme bed positions to determine their effects on the respiratory system. Blood samples would be obtained after the patient had been in a fixed horizontal position for a two hour period. The bed would then be locked in the extreme side-lying position for a two hour period, after which another blood sample would be obtained. A comparative analysis would be done to determine the effects of these positionings on arterial blood gas values.

IMPLICATIONS FOR NURSING

Due to favorable results of a recent multisystem study of 125 patients treated on the Roto-Rest Bed over a 42 month period,[11] this researcher believes that kinetic nursing does indeed reduce the hazards of immobility to all of our bodily systems. This belief was also substantiated by a review of the literature and by clinical experience with kinetically nursed patients. Since kinetic nursing has been shown to reduce the morbidity and mortality associated with immo-

---

11. Barth A. Green, Kathy L. Green, K. J. Klose, Nancy P. Wade, "Kinetic Therapy for Neurological Trauma and Disease: A Review of 125 Patient Experiences," unpublished article, p. 1.

bility, the future implications for nursing are potentially profound.

Summary

The study examined the effects of kinetic nursing on the respiratory systems of immobilized patients by analyzing a series of arterial blood gas values. The convenience sample consisted of ten neurological patients between 17 and 35 years of age who were treated on the Roto-Rest Bed. A series of three arterial blood gas values was obtained at specified time intervals. The PaO_2, $PaCO_2$, and pH were examined to determine the effect of alternating periods of kinesis and akinesis. The hypothesis, that there would be no significant change in immobilized patients' arterial blood gas values when the Roto-Rest Bed is temporarily stopped, was supported. Recommendations included modifications of the methodology to further determine the effect of kinetic nursing in reducing the hazards of immobility.

Bibliography

Brink, Pamela J., and Ward, Marilynn J. *Basic Steps in Planning Nursing Research*. North Scituate, Mass.: Duxbury Press, 1978.

Deitrick, John E., Whedon, Donald, and Shorr, Ephraim. "Effects of Immobilization Upon Various Metabolic and Physiologic Functions of Normal Men." *American Journal of Medicine* 8 (January 1948):3–34.

Ferguson, George A. *Statistical Analysis in Psychology and Education*. New York: McGraw-Hill, 1976.

Green, B. A. "Kinetic Nursing for Spinal Cord Injuries." *Paraplegia Life* (January–February 1976):1–5.

Green, Barth A., Green, Kathy L., Klose, K. J., Wade, Nancy P., "Kinetic Therapy for Neurological Trauma and Disease: A Review of 125 Patient Experiences." Unpublished article:1–15.

Keane, F. X. "Kinetic Nursing." Unpublished article:1–4.

Keane, F. X. "Roto-Rest." *British Medical Journal* 16 (September 1967):731–733.

Miller, Benjamin F., and Keane, Claire. *Encyclopedia and Dictionary of Medicine, Nursing, and Allied Health.* Philadelphia: W. B. Saunders, 1978.

Schimmel, Lawrence, Civetta, Joseph, and Kirby, Robert R. "Treatment of Unilateral Pulmonary Contusion by a New Mechanical Method to Influence Pulmonary Perfusion." *Journal of Critical Care Medicine* (November–December 1977):206–207.

Thompson, Lida F. "The Hazards of Immobility: Effects on Respiratory Function." *American Journal of Nursing* 67 (April 1967):1–17.

Valentin, Lorraine. "Kinetic Nursing and the Roto-Rest Bed." *Orthopedic Nurses' Association Journal* 4 (March 1977):62–65.

Whedon, Donald, Deitrick, John E., Shorr, Ephraim. "Modification of the Effects of Immobilization Upon Metabolic and Physiologic Functions of Normal Men by the Use of an Oscillating Bed." *American Journal of Medicine* 8 (June 1949):684–710.

Appendix

Table 5 Analysis of Variance Design for Each Dependent
Measure (Raw Data)

	T_1		T_2		T_3	
S_1	PaO_2	142	PaO_2	147	PaO_2	134
	$PaCO_2$	42	$PaCO_2$	42	$PaCO_2$	43
	pH	7.41	pH	7.47	pH	7.47
S_2	PaO_2	91	PaO_2	97	PaO_2	85
	$PaCO_2$	40	$PaCO_2$	43	$PaCO_2$	46
	pH	7.53	pH	7.53	pH	7.50
S_3	PaO_2	112	PaO_2	119	PaO_2	116
	$PaCO_2$	29	$PaCO_2$	37	$PaCO_2$	34
	pH	7.44	pH	7.43	pH	7.46
S_4	PaO_2	92	PaO_2	56	PaO_2	72
	$PaCO_2$	38	$PaCO_2$	39	$PaCO_2$	39
	pH	7.41	pH	7.37	pH	7.37
S_5	PaO_2	86	PaO_2	87	PaO_2	87
	$PaCO_2$	37	$PaCO_2$	35	$PaCO_2$	36
	pH	7.37	pH	7.36	pH	7.38
S_6	PaO_2	92	PaO_2	90	PaO_2	91
	$PaCO_2$	34	$PaCO_2$	35	$PaCO_2$	36
	pH	7.34	pH	7.35	pH	7.36
S_7	PaO_2	78	PaO_2	80	PaO_2	80
	$PaCO_2$	37	$PaCO_2$	36	$PaCO_2$	39
	pH	7.32	pH	7.34	pH	7.36
S_8	PaO_2	115	PaO_2	113	PaO_2	118
	$PaCO_2$	39	$PaCO_2$	37	$PaCO_2$	36
	pH	7.46	pH	7.52	pH	7.48
S_9	PaO_2	120	PaO_2	118	PaO_2	124
	$PaCO_2$	47	$PaCO_2$	45	$PaCO_2$	48
	pH	7.36	pH	7.36	pH	7.37
S_{10}	PaO_2	102	PaO_2	102	PaO_2	104
	$PaCO_2$	35	$PaCO_2$	37	$PaCO_2$	39
	pH	7.36	pH	7.40	pH	7.42

Appendix F

ETHICAL CONSIDERATIONS FOR THE PROTECTION OF HUMAN RIGHTS IN RESEARCH

In conducting research on human subjects, nurse researchers must balance the need for knowledge to advance nursing's scientific basis, on the one hand, and the need to protect the research subjects' basic human rights, on the other.

Researchers working with human subjects must always remember that their subjects are real people with needs and wants and not just numbers on a piece of paper. To this end, codes of ethics for human subject research have been developed to insure the subjects' dignity and safety and the worthiness of human subject research projects.

The 1975 *Human Rights Guidelines for Nurses in Clinical and Other Research,* published by the American Nurses' Association, outline the responsibilities for nurses in practice, education, and research in safeguarding the rights of others. We recommend that you become familiar with these guidelines as well as the material in this discussion.

The subjects of research include patients and outpatients, persons who are donors of organs and tissues, research volunteers, as well as volunteers with limited freedom —those who are members of groups vulnerable to exploitation. Included in this classification are prisoners, residents in institutions for the mentally ill and mentally retarded, and military personnel.[1]

As a result of the increasing awareness of ethical decision-making in human subject research over the years, most institutions sponsoring human subject research have a review group or committee whose responsibility it is to insure that researchers do not engage in unethical behavior. "Membership on the review committee should be representative of all occupational groups (including practicing nurses) whose members are likely to be involved either directly or indirectly in the implementation of the activities or projects undertaken." [2]

---

1. American Nurses' Association, *Human Rights Guidelines for Nurses in Clinical and Other Research,* Code No. D-465M (Kansas City: The Association, July 1975), p. 5.
2. Ibid., p. 8.

Further, state and federal laws and agencies have been set up to insure that ethical research standards are met. No researcher applying for a federal grant can avoid the scrutiny of his or her research proposal, or the provision of formal assurance for maintaining proper ethical standards.

The greatest concern in human subject research is the protection of the subject's right of self determination by the assurance of informed consent. This means that the subject must be made fully aware of the study and agree to participate in it. The need for this type of agreement may seem self evident, but a large number of studies have been carried out without the participants' consent. A glaring and tragic example of such research in the United States is the study of males with venereal disease carried out during the 1930s. In this study, subjects thought that they had received treatment for venereal disease. Treatment was withheld from a sample of the population, however, while the remainder received treatment. The so-called researchers then intended to follow the subjects through the remainder of their lives to determine the effects of venereal disease. At the time of this writing, the survivors of this "experiment" are still being sought, and large amounts of monetary compensation are being given to them and their survivors. There was no excuse for not obtaining their consent initially; the cost in suffering and disability can never be justified.

Essentially, informed consent consists of the following six elements:

1. An understandable explanation of the procedures and techniques to be followed is required, along with the identification of experimental procedures and techniques. Fulfilling this requirement is difficult. As pointed out in Chapter 9, the awareness of subjects about the nature of the research or experiment may affect the experiment. There are those who suggest that a researcher cannot get a true random sample of a population, in fact, because consenting to an experiment automatically means that the subjects in the experimental study are different from those subjects who refused to participate.

2. An explanation is required of the potential risks and discomforts to the subject as a result of the experiment. Will the subject be exposed to a potentially harmful situation? Withholding medication or treatment may cause physical or psychological distress to the subject. Further, withholding treatment may actually expose the subject to physical risk. Each subject must know what the potential hazards are. Further, the right of personal privacy and dignity for each subject must be assured.

3. Subjects should be told what benefits are to be expected. This can be a broad explanation; it may be the basis for an appeal to the subject's altruism, or it may be merely a simple explanation. The intent of many experiments is to improve the human condition. By providing different treatments to research subjects, treatment modalities may improve. Each time a new treatment is tried, it is usually believed to be more effective than existing treatments.

4. Subjects must be told of alternative procedures that would be advantageous to the subject. For example, in the case of the use of an experimental drug, subjects should be aware that other, already proven drugs, may aid in the treatment while the experimental drug may do nothing at all. Subjects must also be informed if benefits are to be withheld from them.

5. Researchers must be willing to answer any question that the subjects may have about the experimental procedures. Most subjects want to know what is happening and why it is happening. The aloof professional who fails to explain things to the patient can potentially do more harm than good. In a research situation, subjects must be informed of what is happening if they request such information.

6. Subjects must be made aware that they can withdraw from the research investigation at any time. Researchers cannot compel or coerce subjects to continue in any project against their will.

It is essential that the researcher be able to document that he or she has obtained the informed consent of the subject. Such consent is best obtained on a written form

stating that the subject has willingly entered into the research project, and is aware of the risks, procedures and
benefits involved. The following form might be used:

> I _____ (subject) do agree to participate in a re-
> search/experimental study concerning _____. This
> project may expose me to _____ risks and attendant
> discomforts.
>
> I am aware that _____ might be advantageous
> to me in the treatment of my conditions instead of the
> experimental treatment.
>
> I may ask any questions about the procedures and
> treatments taking place and my questions must be an-
> swered honestly and fully.
>
> I am free to withdraw this consent and discontinue
> participation in this research project at any time.

_____
Signature of subject

Oral consents are also valid, but should be witnessed by
a third party for the protection of both the researcher and
the subject. In the event that the potential subjects are not
able to give informed consent because of mental or physical
disabilities, or are below the legal age of consent, the researcher must gain the consent of a legally authorized guard-
ian or next of kin.

Upon completion of the research investigation involving
human subjects, the researcher has the obligation to remove
any harmful aftereffects and to follow through on any com-
mitments made to the subject, including the provision of
any study results that have been promised. Anonymity of the
subjects must be maintained as well as the confidentiality of
the subjects' responses.

Finally, nurses have the professional obligation to become knowledgeable participants in health care practice and
research, and to assure that they involve themselves in institutional policy making and review activities:

Knowledge about the changing scope of nursing responsibility and the emerging ethical issues affecting all practitioners in health care today is a necessary requirement for professional nursing practice in which accountability for the protection of human rights of consumers is accepted.[3]

3. Ibid., p. 11.

Comments

4. Reference format:
   a. Citation (footnote) references
      are listed in consistent and
      correct format.
   b. Bibliographic entries are listed
      in consistent and correct format.

Further Notes on Writing a Research Proposal

Now that you have a tentative draft of the major sections of your research proposal, reread the draft to be sure you have a logical development of ideas within each section and throughout the proposal. You may want to exchange yours with a classmate and use the evaluation guidelines.

In addition to the criteria listed in the guidelines, in the procedure part of the data collection section you may want to include a timetable for the various steps to be followed in carrying out the research project, as well as an estimate of the expenses associated with the research project. Research proposals written for funding require that a budget of projected expenses be included. Guidelines for funding such proposals are very specific regarding the budget information to be included.

The title of your proposal should accurately reflect the relationship between the variables being studied and the population of the study. The title can be most easily formulated from the information in the purpose of the study section, and should reflect this purpose well enough to communicate it to others. Ask yourself if someone reading the title in an index would know what your study is about. A well formulated proposal title can usually serve as the title for the final report of the study.

Remember to use the future tense and to refer to yourself as "the investigator" or "the researcher." In terms of proposal length, rarely does a final proposal written by a beginning researcher exceed twenty to twenty-five typed, double-spaced pages, including bibliography and appendices.

Appendix H

**GUIDELINES FOR EVALUATING A
RESEARCH REPORT**

As an aid in estimating the study's general level of acceptability, our students have found it helpful to tally the *Yes* responses and divide them by the total possible responses *(Yes/Total)*. This gives you a percentage that can be used to estimate the study's *general* level of acceptability. One major caution, however: some components of the guidelines are more critical than others. This general evaluation method must be accompanied by logic and judgment. For example, an inadequate title is not as critical to the study's acceptability as inadequate interpretation of data. Likewise, if the whole data collection section is unacceptable, the study's findings are not valid.

Guidelines for Evaluating a Research Report

Yes   No   N/A *

A. *The Problem*
1. The problem is clearly identified.
2. The problem is researchable (data can be collected and analyzed).
3. It is feasible to conduct research on the problem.
4. The problem is significant to nursing.
5. Background information on the problem is presented.

B. *The Review of the Literature*
1. The review is relevant to the study.
2. The review is adequate in relation to the problem.
3. Sources are current.
4. Documentation of sources is clear and complete.
5. The relationship of the problem to previous research is clear.
6. There is a range of opinions and varying points of view about the problem.

Yes   No N/A *

7. The organization of the review is
   logical.
8. The review concludes with a brief
   summary of the literature and its
   implications for the problem.

C. *Theoretical or Conceptual Framework*
   1. Is applicable to the research.
   2. Is clearly developed.
   3. Is useful for clarifying pertinent
      concepts and relationships.

D. *Statement of the Purpose of the Study*
   1. The statement form is appropriate
      for the study: declarative
      statement, question, hypothesis(es).
   2. The statement form is clear as to:
      a. what the researcher plans to do
      b. where the data will be collected
      c. from whom the data will be
         collected
   3. Each hypothesis states an expected
      relationship or difference between
      two (2) variables.
   4. There is a clear empirical or
      theoretical rationale for each
      hypothesis.

E. *Definition of Terms*
   1. Relevant terms are clearly defined,
      either directly or operationally.

F. *Data Collection*
   1. Study Subjects
      a. The target population is clearly
         described.
      b. The sample size and major
         characteristics are appropriate
         (the sample is representative).
      c. The method for choosing the
         sample is appropriate.

Yes   No   N/A *

    d. The sample size is adequate for
the problem being investigated.

2. Data Collection Instruments

    a. Instruments are appropriate for
problem and method.

    b. Rationale for choosing
instruments is discussed.

    c. Each instrument is described as
to purpose, content, strengths and
weaknesses.

    d. Instrument validity is discussed.

    e. Instrument reliability is
discussed.

    f. If the instrument was developed
for the study:

        1. Rationale for development is
discussed

        2. Procedures in development are
discussed

        3. Reliability is discussed

        4. Validity is discussed

3. Procedures

    a. The research approach is
appropriate.

    b. Steps in the data collection
procedure are described clearly
and concisely.

    c. The data collection procedure is
appropriate for the study.

    d. Protection of human rights is
assured.

    e. The study is replicable from the
information provided.

    f. Appropriate limitations of the
study are stated.

    g. Significant assumptions are
stated.

Yes   No   N/A *

G. *Data Analysis*

  1. The choice of statistical procedures is appropriate.

  2. Statistical procedures are correctly applied to the data.

  3. Tables, charts, graphs are clear and well labeled.

  4. Tables, charts, graphs are pertinent.

  5. Tables, charts, graphs reflect reported findings.

  6. Tables, charts, graphs are clearly discussed in the text.

H. *Conclusions and Recommendations*

  1. Results are discussed in relation to the study's purpose.

  2. Results are discussed in relation to the conceptual or theoretical framework.

  3. Interpretations are based on the data.

  4. Generalizations are warranted by the results.

  5. Conclusions are based on the data.

  6. Conclusions are clearly stated.

  7. Recommendations are plausible and relevant.

I. *Summary*

  1. The summary restates the problem.

  2. The summary restates the methodology.

  3. The summary restates the major findings and conclusions.

  4. The summary is clear and concise.

J. *Other Considerations*

  1. The investigator(s) is qualified.

  2. The title is appropriate, accurately reflecting the problem.

                                                    Yes   No N/A *
3. The article is well organized and
   flows logically.
4. Grammar, sentence structure, and
   punctuation are correct.
5. References and bibliography are
   accurate and complete.
* Not Applicable

Conclusions regarding the general level of acceptability of
the study:

Glossary

Applied research   research conducted to generate new knowledge that can be applied in practical settings without undue delay.

Assumptions   underlying principles based on the belief of their correctness in a research design.

Basic research   research designed to formulate theory rather than be utilized for immediate application.

Case study   an in-depth study of individuals or small groups

Chi-square (χ^2)   a statistical technique used to determine if observed values differ from expected values.

Concept   a single idea (often one word) which represents several related component ideas (i.e., "grief").

Conceptual framework   discussion of the relationship of concepts that underly the study problem and support the rationale (reason) for conducting the study.

Confounding variables   variables that may interfere with the direct causal relationship of independent to dependent variables.

Content validity   a method for determining validity of a measuring instrument that utilizes consensus of a judge panel of experts. The panel agrees that a measuring instrument measures what it is said to measure.

Control group   the group in which the experimental treatment is not introduced.

Correlation   the quantifiable relationship between two or more variables.

Criterion variable   a preestablished measure of success. Sometimes called the dependent variable.

Cross-sectional survey   a research technique in which data are collected at a certain point in time.

Data   plural of *datum*.

Datum   a unit of information.

Delphi technique   a research methodology used to predict or emphasize the main concerns of a group.

Dependent variable   the variable that changes as the independent variable is manipulated by the researcher. Sometimes called the criterion variable.

Descriptive research   research approach that is present oriented and describes current attitudes or events.

Empirical evidence   evidence gathered to generate new knowledge. It must be rooted in objective reality and gathered directly or indirectly through the human senses.

Experimental research   research approach in which the independent variable(s) is manipulated under controlled conditions to determine the effect on the dependent variable(s).

Exploratory study (pilot study)   a preliminary study used to determine strengths and weaknesses of a planned project. May also be the basis of future studies.

External criticism   the evaluation of the validity of historical data.

Extraneous variable   uncontrolled variables outside of the purpose of the study that influence the study's results.

Face validity   a subjective method for determining validity of a measuring instrument. It is determined by inspection of the items to see that the instrument contains important items that measure the variables being studied.

Frequency distribution   the arrangement of the scores or values of characteristics in a systematic way.

Hawthorne effect   term used to describe the psychological reactions to the presence of the investigator, or to special treatment during a research study, which tend to alter the responses of the subject.

Historical research   research approach that deals with what has happened in the past and how those happenings affect the present.

H₀ *see* Null hypothesis.

Hypothesis a statement of the predicted relationship between the variables under study; an educated or calculated guess by the researcher. It is the testable component of the research; *hypotheses* is the plural form.

Independent variable the variable that is purposely manipulated or changed by the researcher (also termed the Manipulated Variable).

Inference information gathered from a sample is generalized to a population.

Internal criticism the evaluation of the reliability of historical data.

Interval data data based on a scale that has equal intervals and a zero starting point.

Interview verbal questioning of respondents by the investigator in order to collect data. Requires interaction between people.

Level of significance the probability level used to reject the null hypothesis.

Likert scale a scale for rating attitudes in which each statement usually has five possible responses: Strongly Agree, Agree, Uncertain, Disagree, Strongly Disagree.

Longitudinal survey a research technique in which data are collected from the same subjects over a period of time.

Mean the arithmetic average.

Measures of central tendency *see* Mean, Median, Mode, Standard deviation. These show how measurements cluster about the mean.

Median the number above which fifty percent of the observations fall.

MEDLARS *(Medical Literature Analysis and Retrieval System)* the computerized literature retrieval service of the National Library of Medicine.

MEDLINE a computerized data base that references bio-medical journal articles.

Mode the most frequently occurring score or number value.

Nominal data data that can be separated into only mutually exclusive categories.

Normal curve a theoretical bell shaped curve with most measurements clustered about the center and few measurements at the extreme ends.

Null hypothesis (H_0) the most commonly used way of stating the relationship between the variables being studied. The null hypothesis is stated as "there is no statistically significant difference between the experimental and control group."

Nursing research research conducted to answer questions, or to find solutions to problems, specifically related to nursing. It has the purpose of developing an organized body of scientific knowledge unique to nursing. Also a nursing journal.

Observation watching and noting actions and reactions.

Operational definition the researcher's definition of a term that provides a description of the method for studying the concept by citing the necessary operations (manipulations and observations) to be used.

Opinionnaire a questionnaire designed to elicit opinions.

Ordinal data data that may be ordered, but for which there is no zero starting point, and the intervals between datum are not equal. Big, bigger, biggest are ordinal data.

Pearson r Pearson product–moment correlation coefficient. A frequently used correlation statistic. r's range from -1 to $+1$.

Pilot study *see* Exploratory study.

Population *see* Target population.

Population element a single unit or member of the target population.

Primary source a source that presents original data, not interpretive or hearsay information.

Projective techniques techniques of psychological testing which require the subjects to respond to an ambiguous situation.

Questionnaire a paper and pencil data collection instrument which is completed by the study subjects themselves to elicit their attitudes or feelings.

r *see* Pearson r.

Random sample *see* Simple random sample or Stratified random sample.

Range the distribution of scores from lowest to highest. The high score minus the low score gives the range.

Rating scale a scale that allows respondents to make a qualitative judgment. Rating scales yield ordinal data.

Reliability the degree to which a measuring instrument obtains consistent results when it is reused.

Replication repeating a study using the same study design but different study subjects.

Research a scientific process of inquiry and/or experimentation that involves purposeful, systematic and rigorous collection, analysis and interpretation of data in order to gain new knowledge, or add to the existing body of scientific knowledge.

Sample a smaller part of the target population selected in such a way that the individuals in the sample represent (as nearly as possible) the characteristics of the target population.

Sampling process of selecting a sample from the target population.

Sampling unit *see* Population element.

Scientific method an orderly process that utilizes the principles of science, and requires the use of certain sequential steps to acquire dependable information in the solving of problems.

Secondary source an interpretive or hearsay source.

Serendipity unplanned and unexpected discovery of significant results in a research study.

Simple random sample a probability sample in which the

required number of sampling units is selected at random from the population in such a manner that each population element has an equal chance (probability) of being selected.

Spurious correlations correlations that yield high relationship values, but no relationship exists.

Standard deviation the general indicator of dispersion from the mean.

Statistics the techniques used to assemble, to describe, and to make inferences from numerical data.

Statistical inference statistical analysis that permits conclusions to be drawn about a population based upon examination of only a portion (sample) of the population.

Stratified random sample a variation of the simple random sample in which the target population is divided into two or more strata (categories of the characteristic), and a simple random sample is then taken from each stratum (category).

Structured interview an interview that has a set series of questions.

Student's test *see* t test.

Survey research collection of data about present conditions directly from the study subjects, usually by questionnaire or interview.

Symbols those signs used to substitute for whole words or concepts, such as χ^2 for chi–square or r for Pearson product–moment correlation coefficient.

Target population the total group of individual people or things meeting the designated set of criteria of interest to the researcher.

t test a statistical measure to determine differences between the means of two groups.

Tests of significance statistical tests utilized to determine differences between groups.

Theoretical framework discussion of one theory or interrelated theories being tested in order to support the rationale (reason) for conducting the study.

Theory a set of statements—called propositions—that are stated in such a way as to form a logically interrelated deductive system. Used to summarize existing knowledge, and explain and/or predict phenomena and their relationships.

Unstructured interview an interview that has a general framework for eliciting data but does not have a fixed pattern of questions.

Validity the extent to which a data-gathering instrument measures what it is supposed to measure by obtaining data relevant to what is being measured.

Variable a multivalued entity. The attribute or characteristic under study that varies along some dimension.

χ^2 *see* Chi–Square.

Index